AF255591

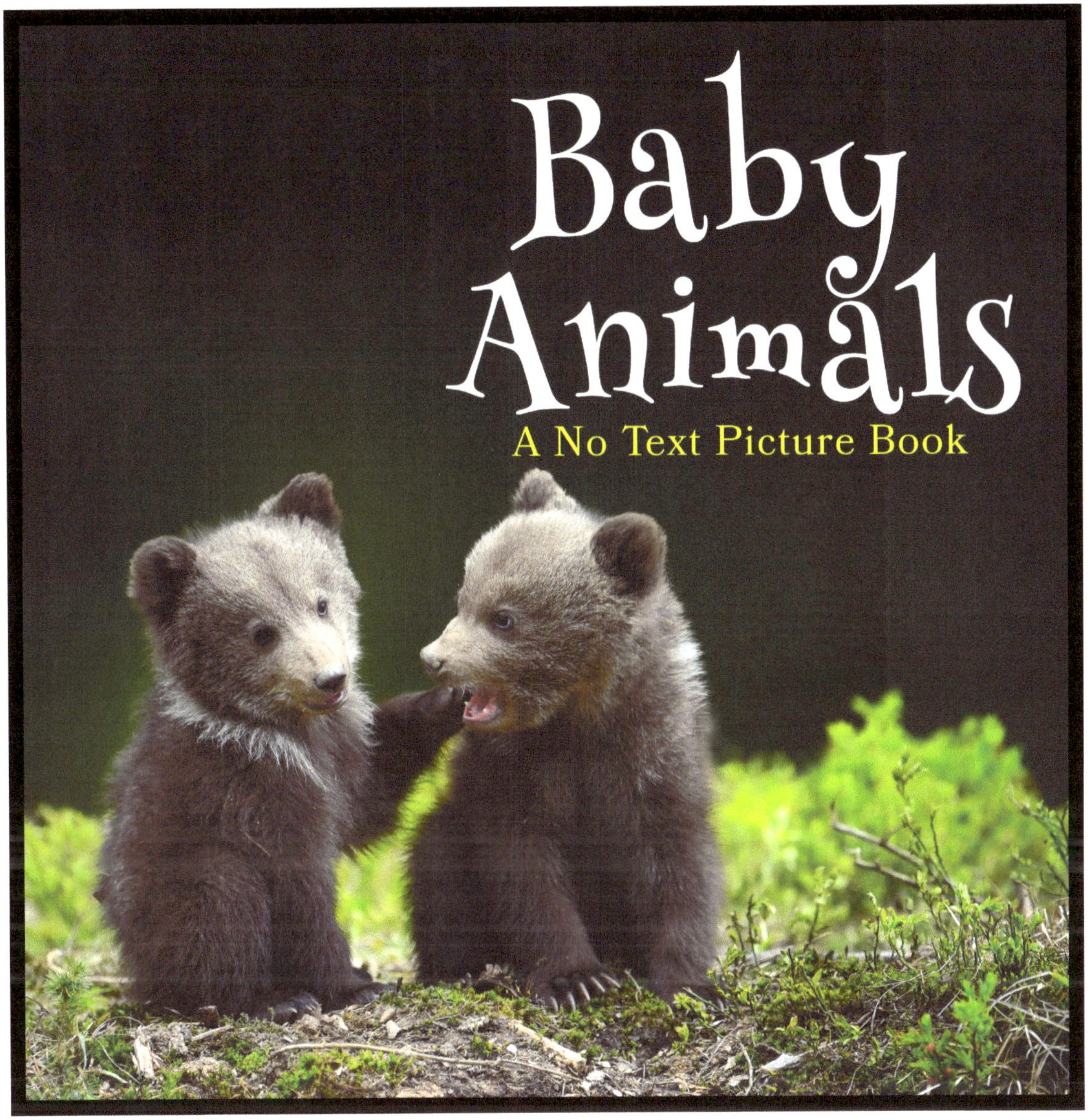

# Baby Animals

## A No Text Picture Book

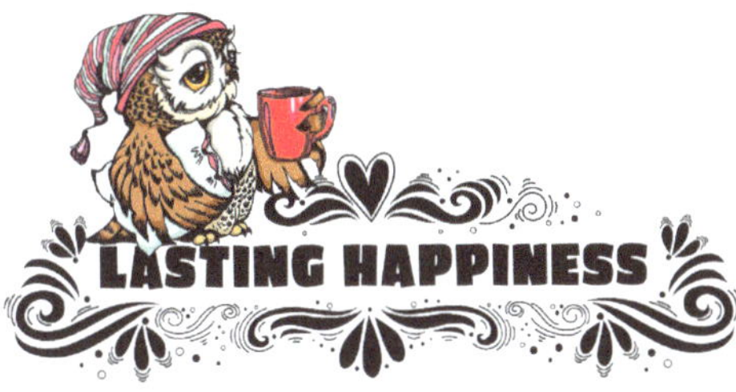



ISBN: 978-1-990181-69-6

To:

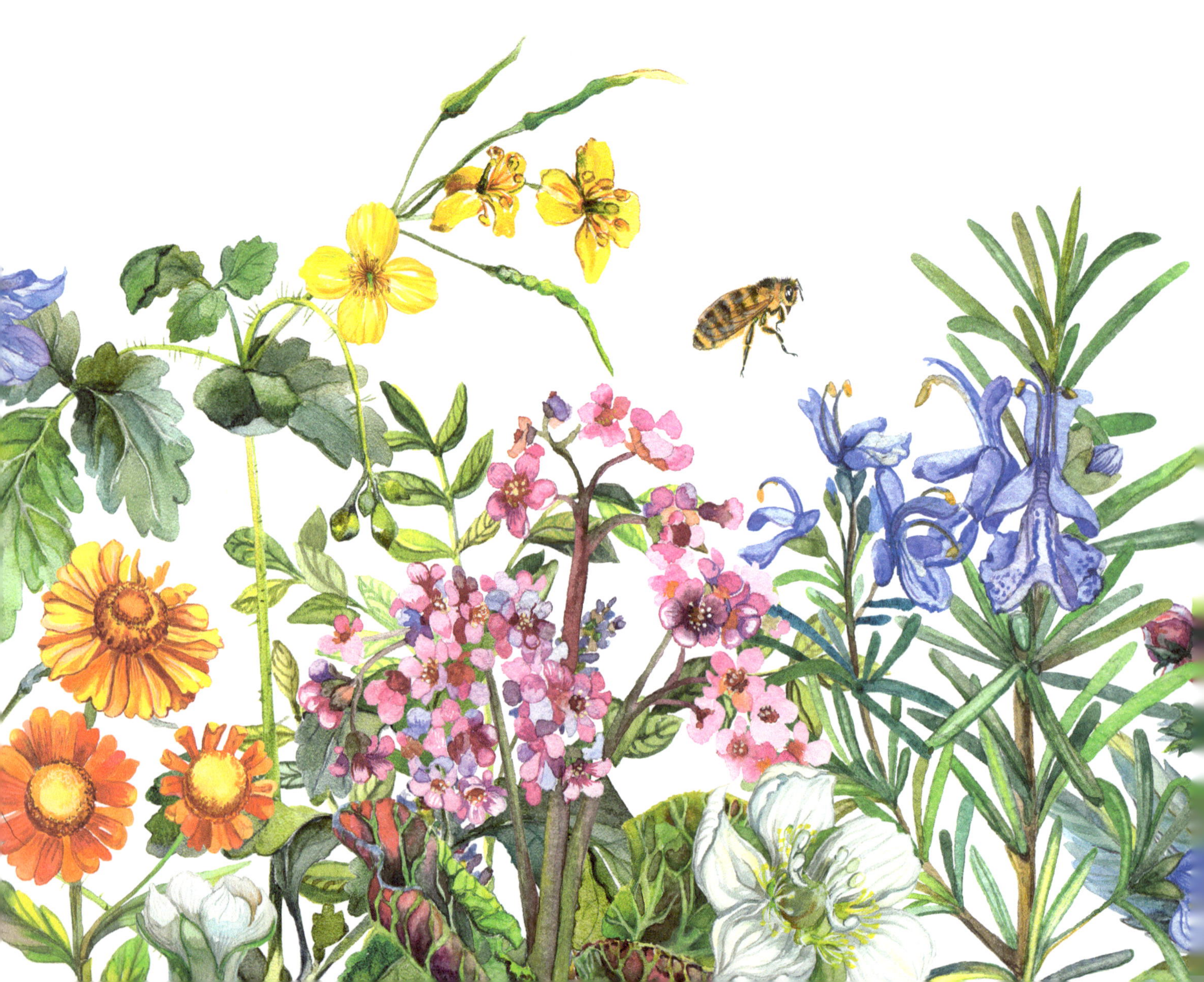

FROM:


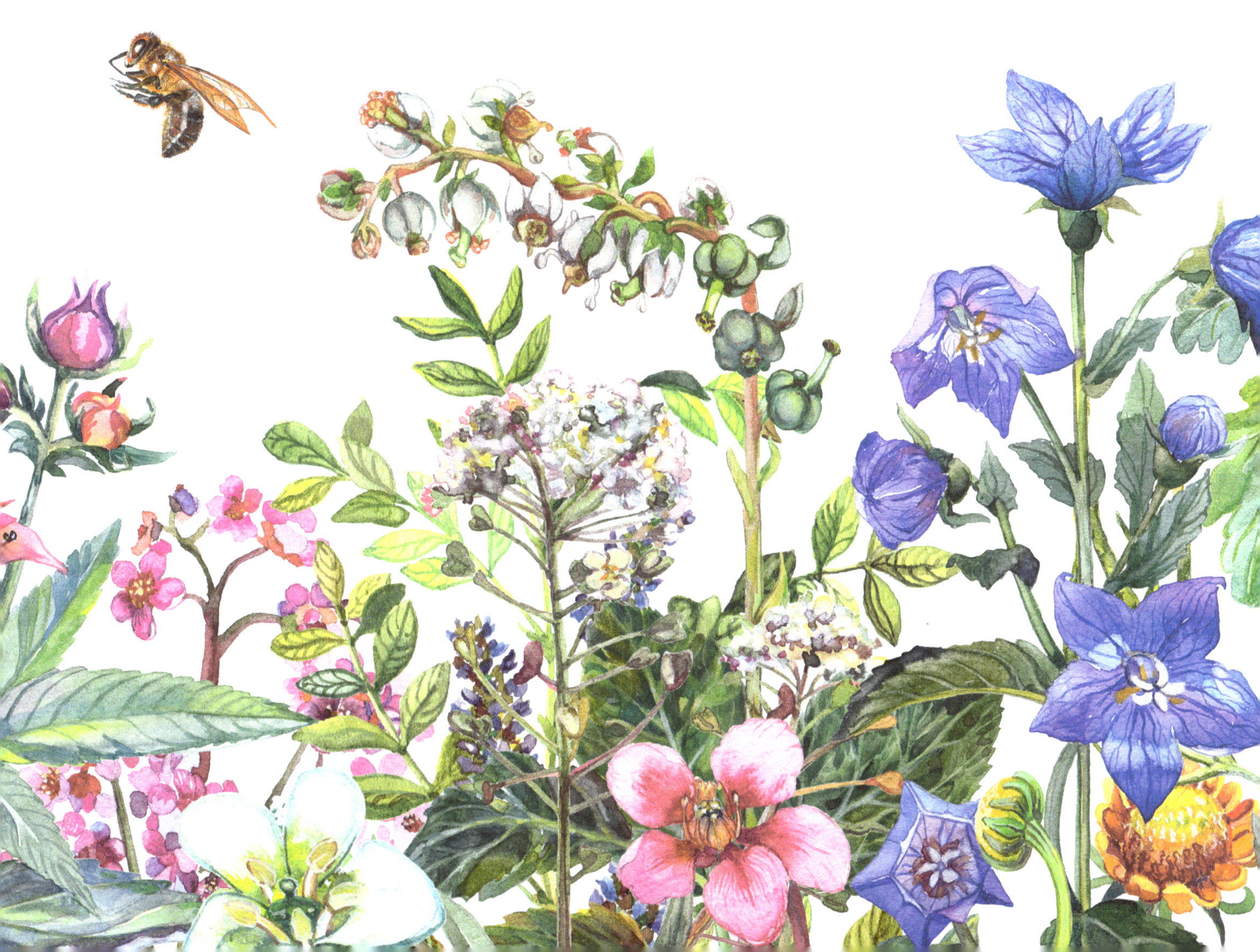

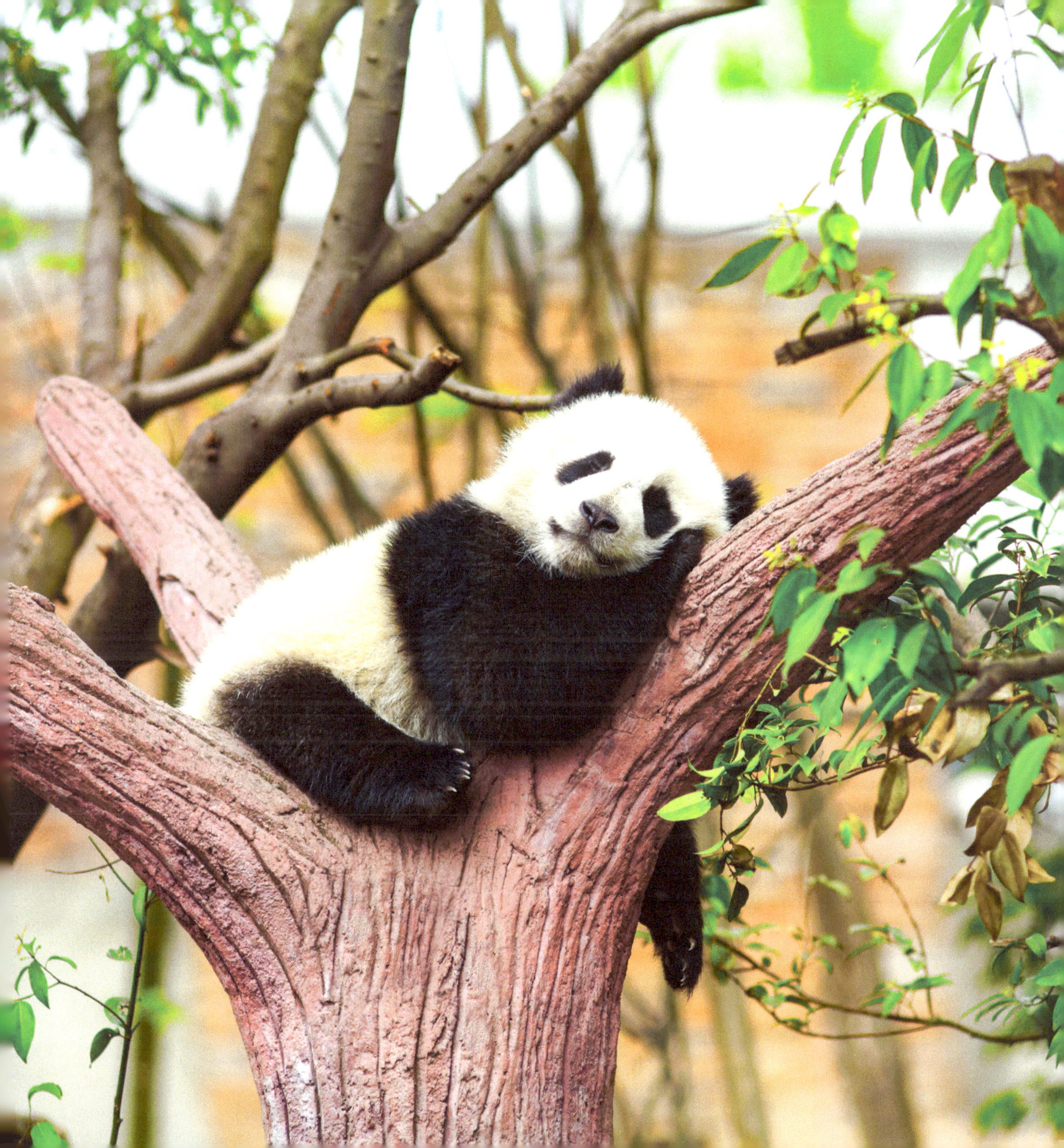

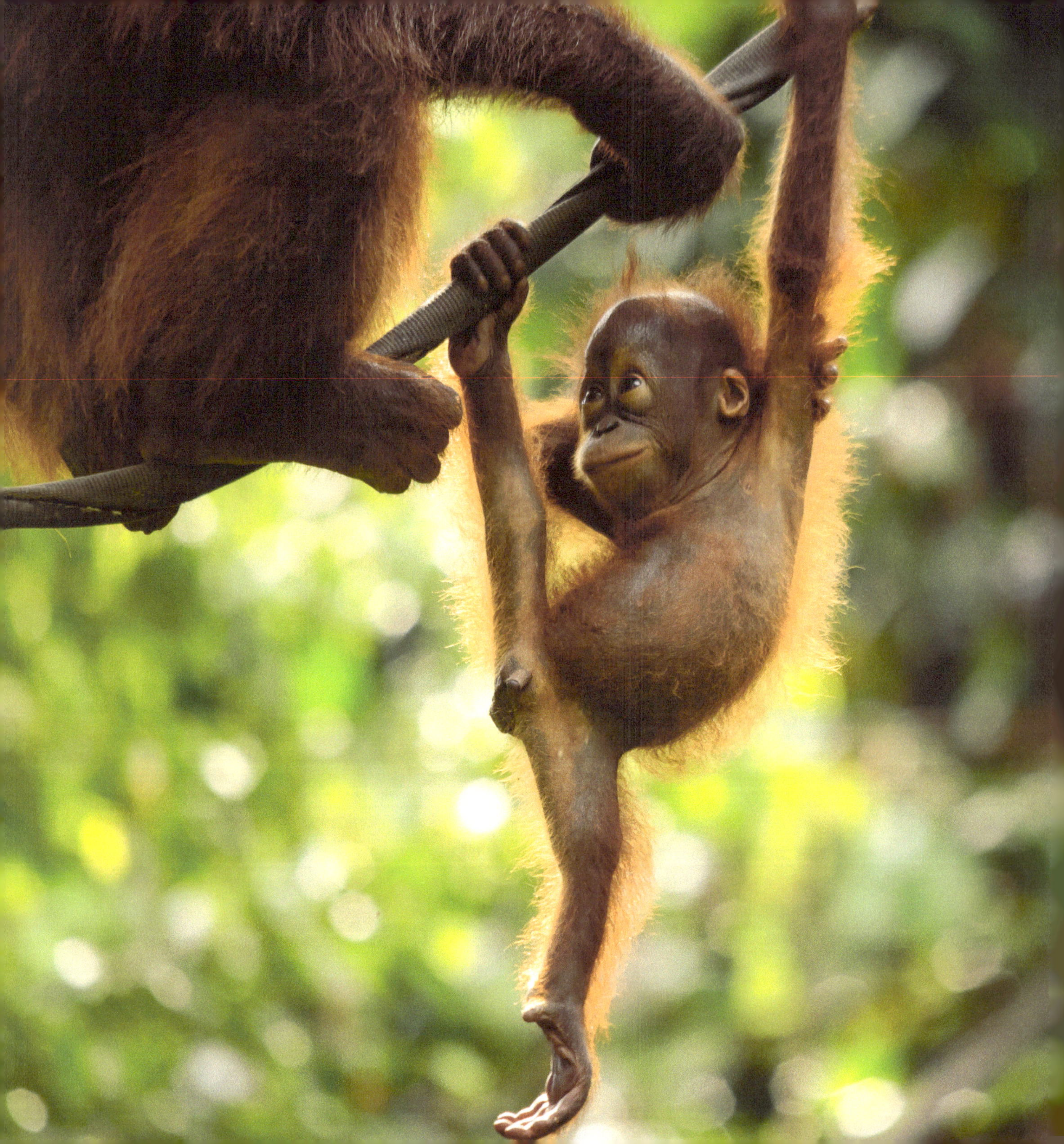

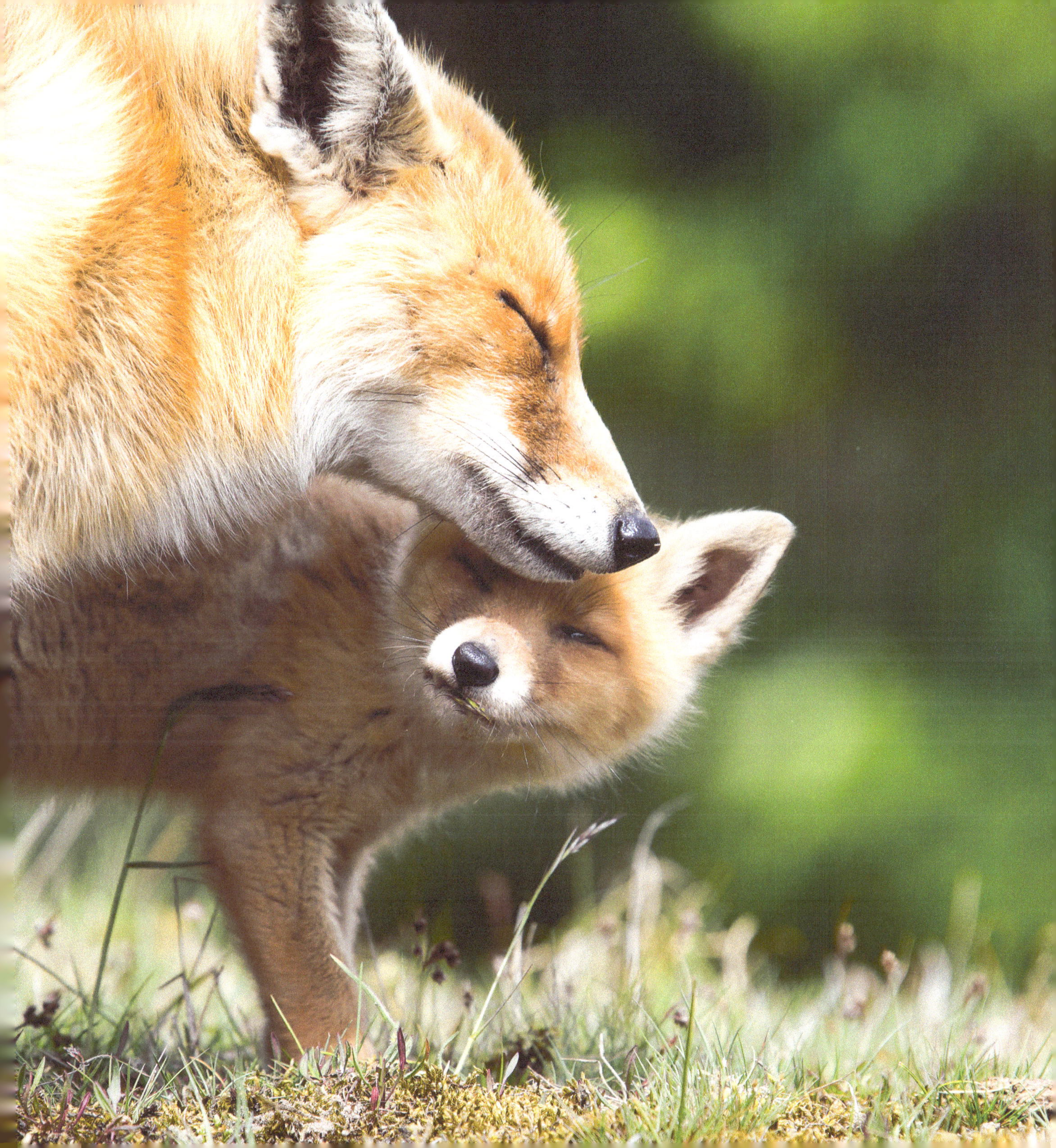

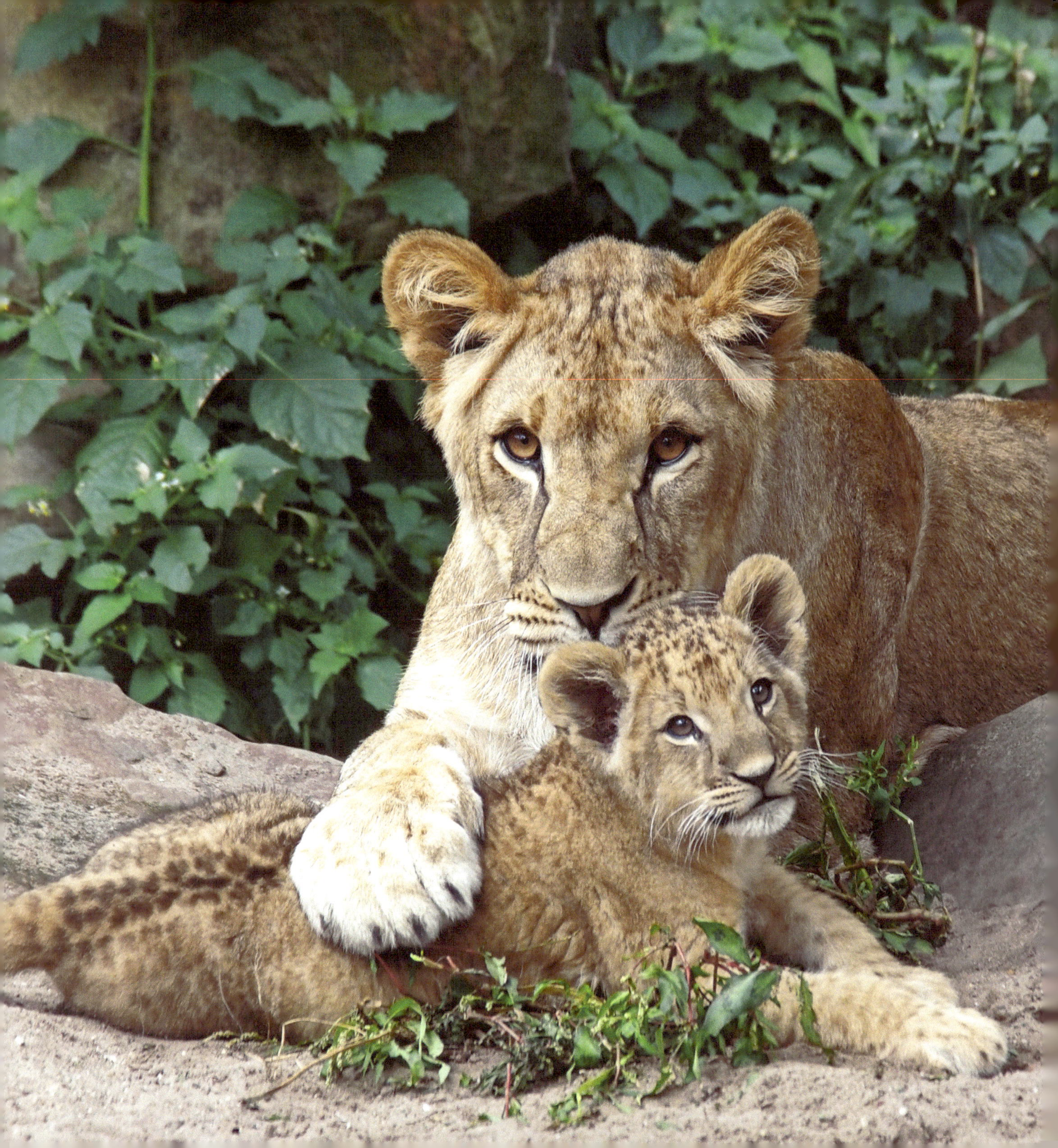

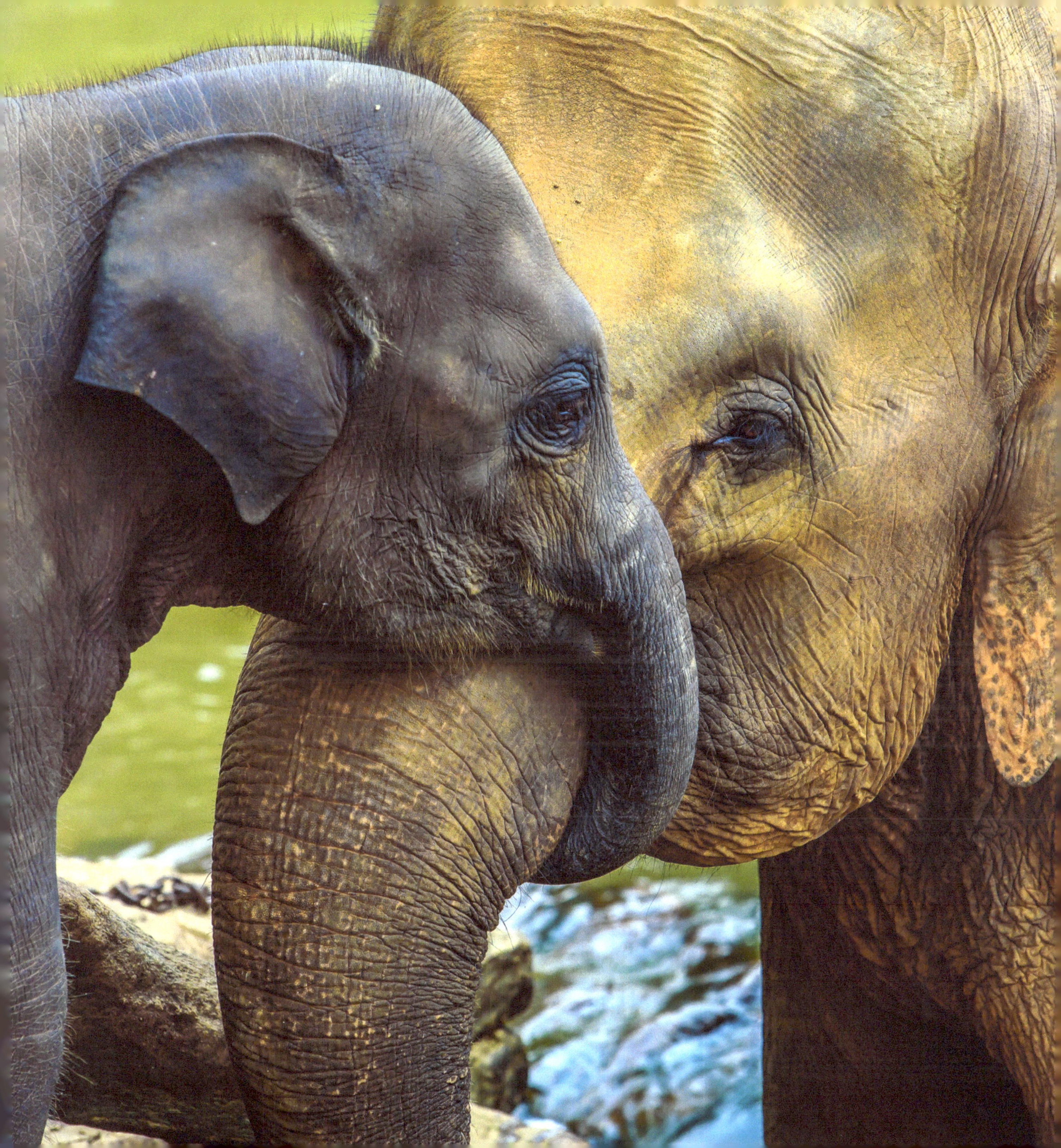

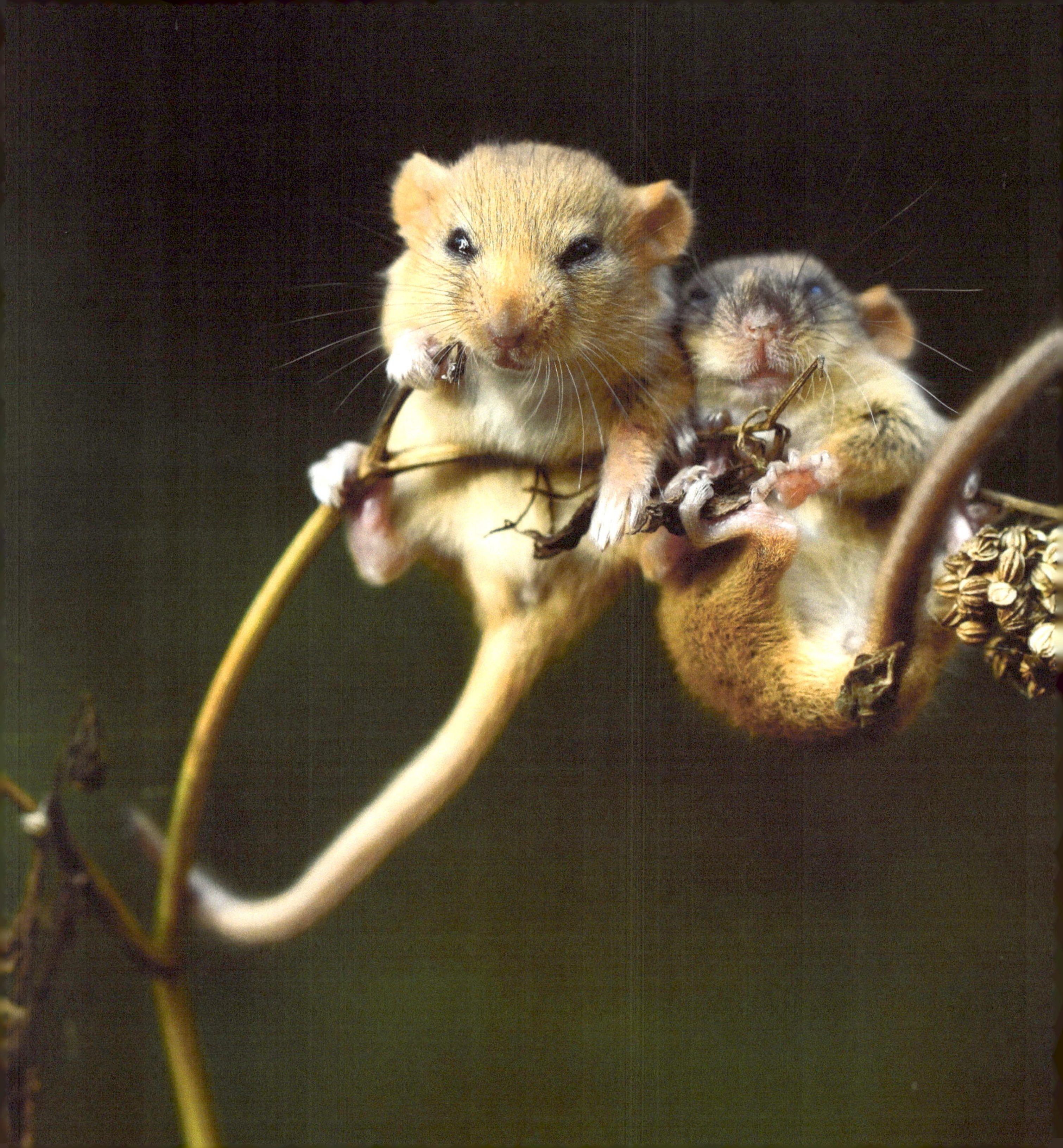

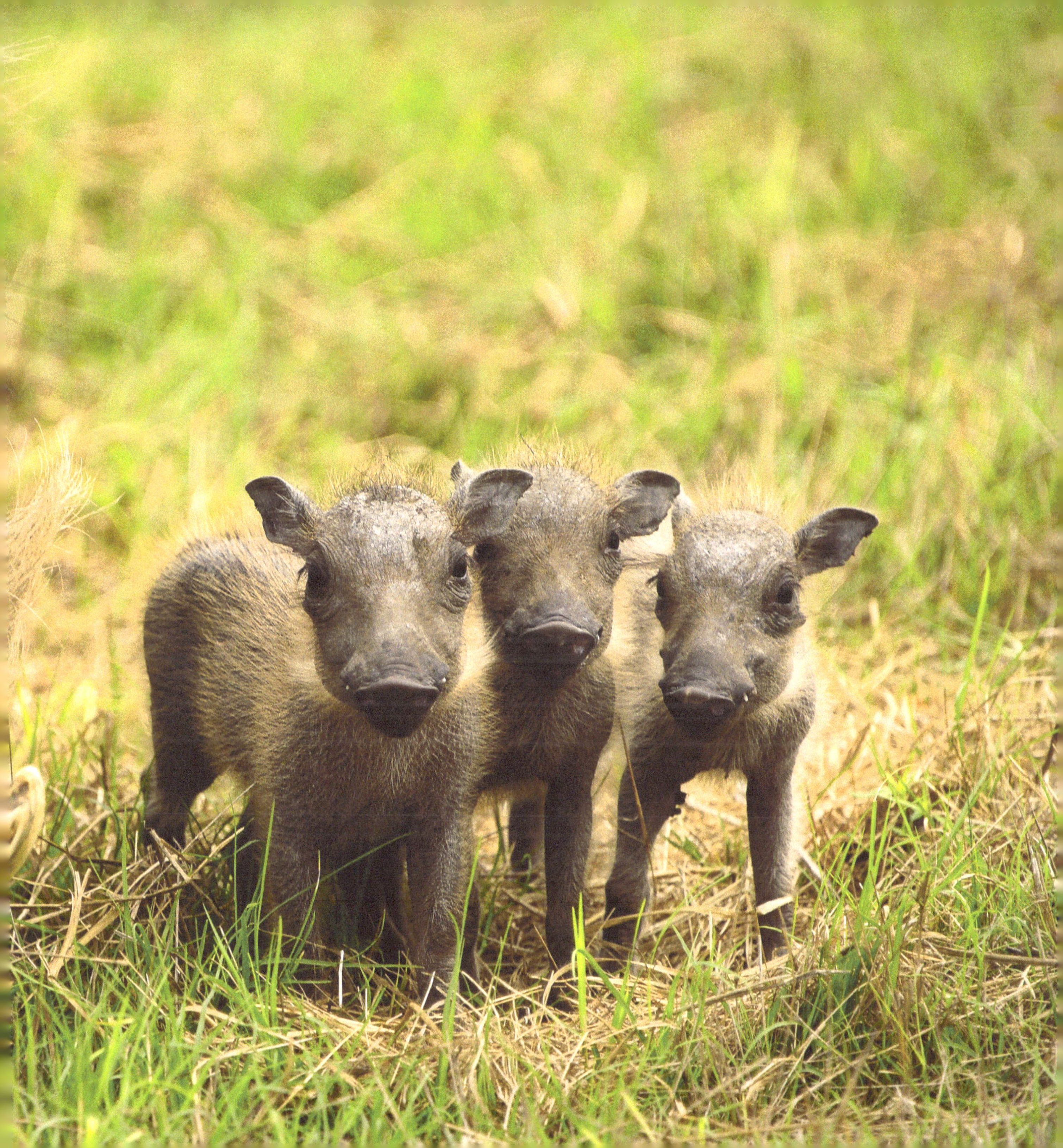

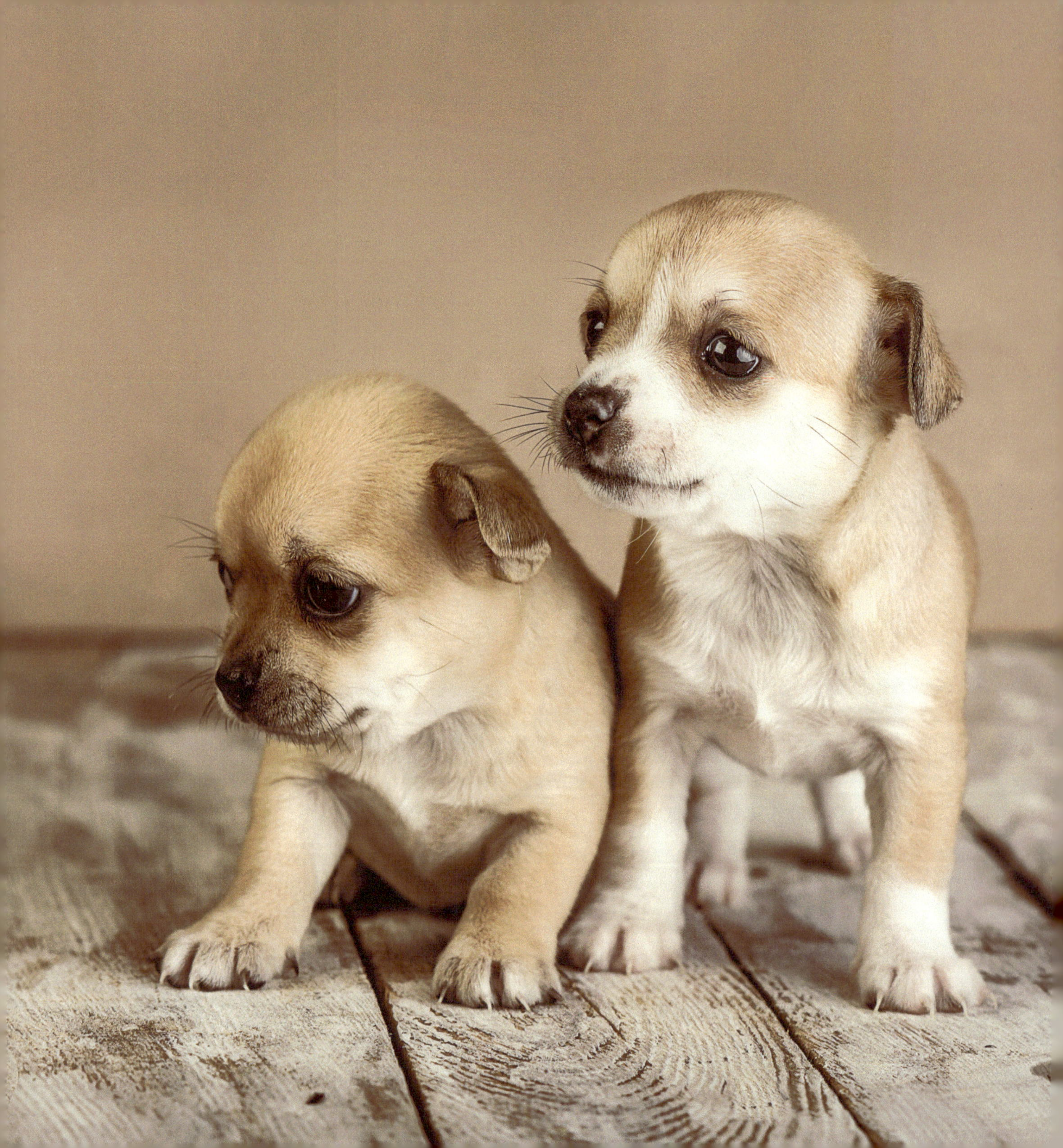

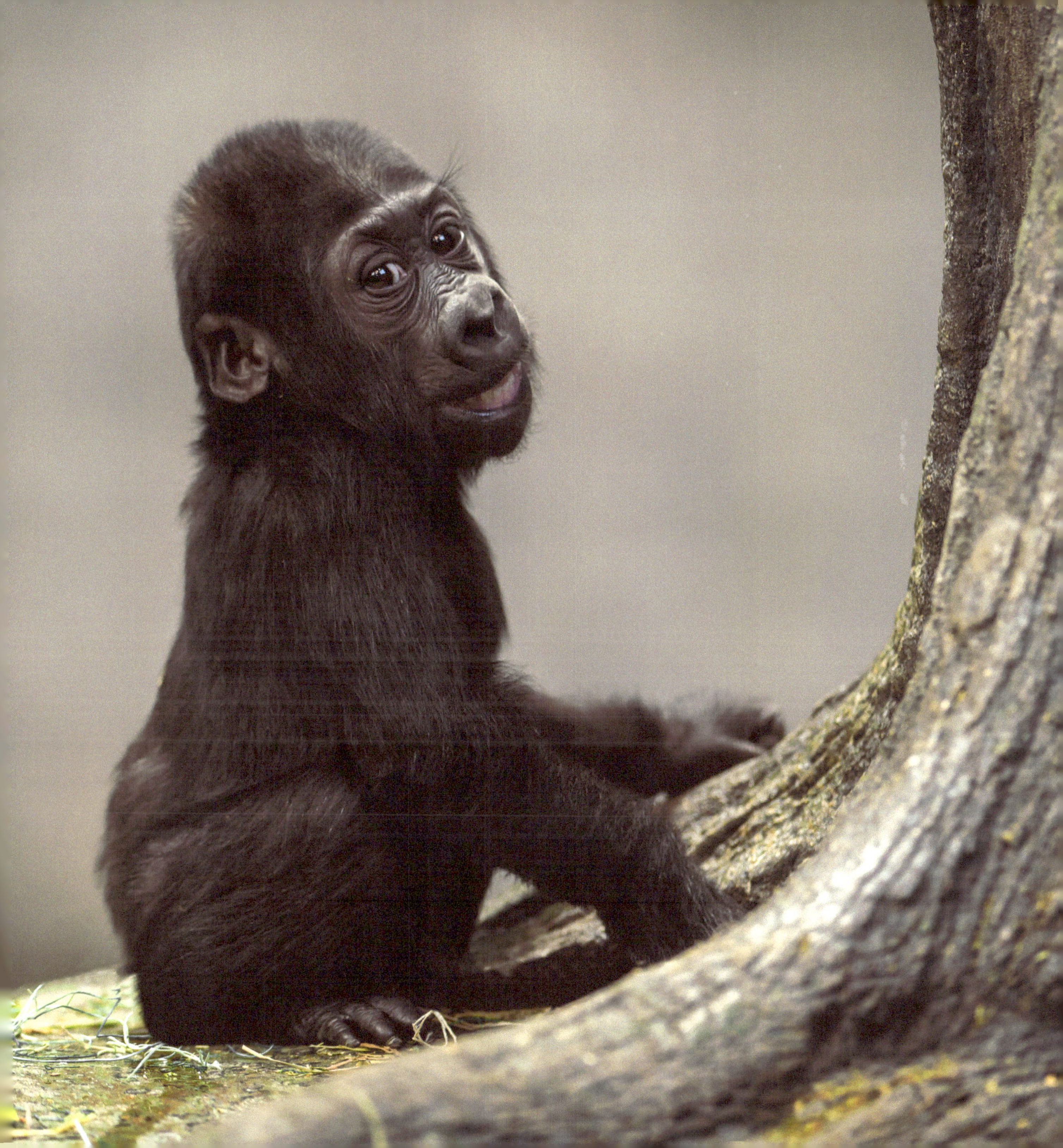

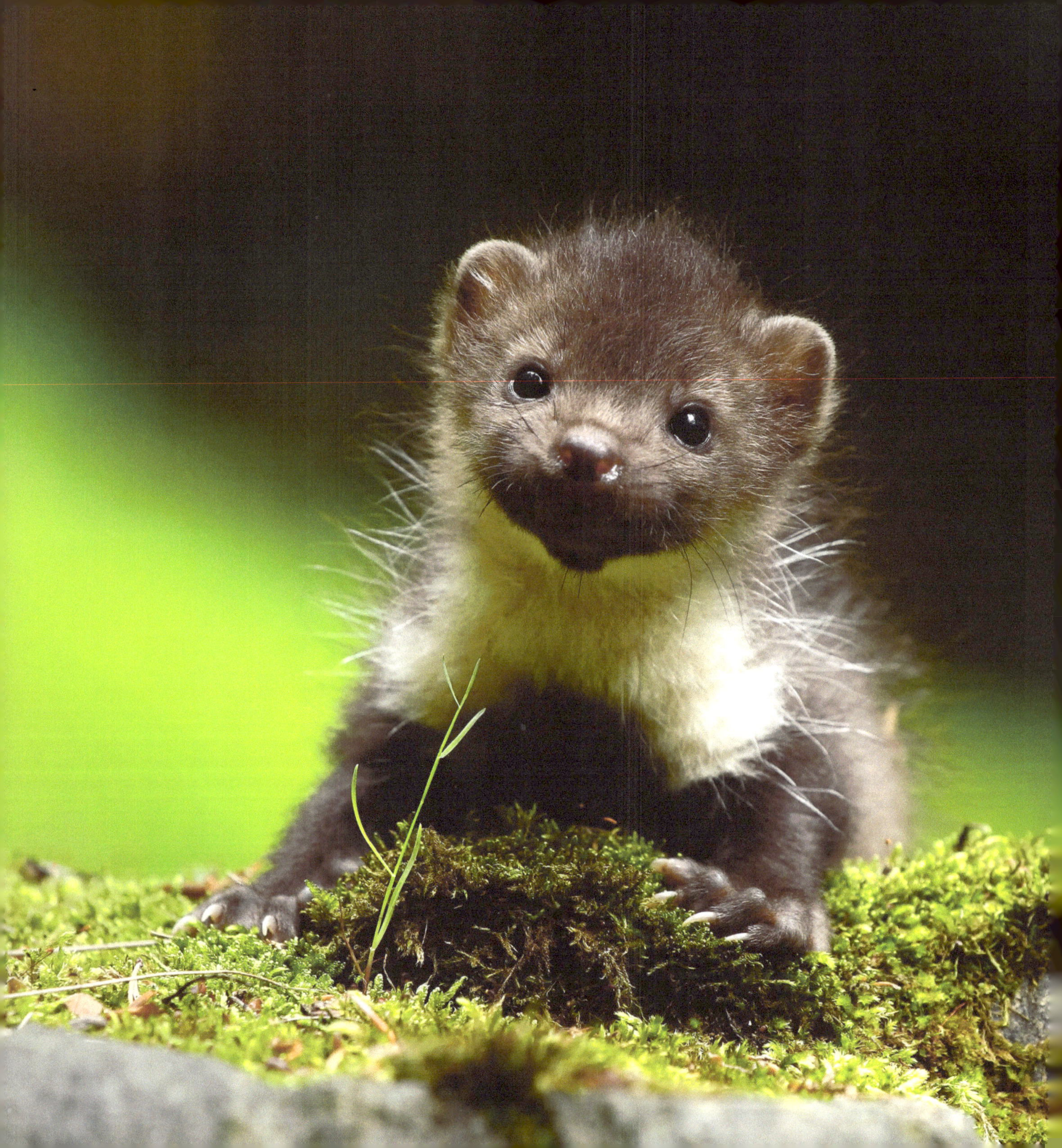

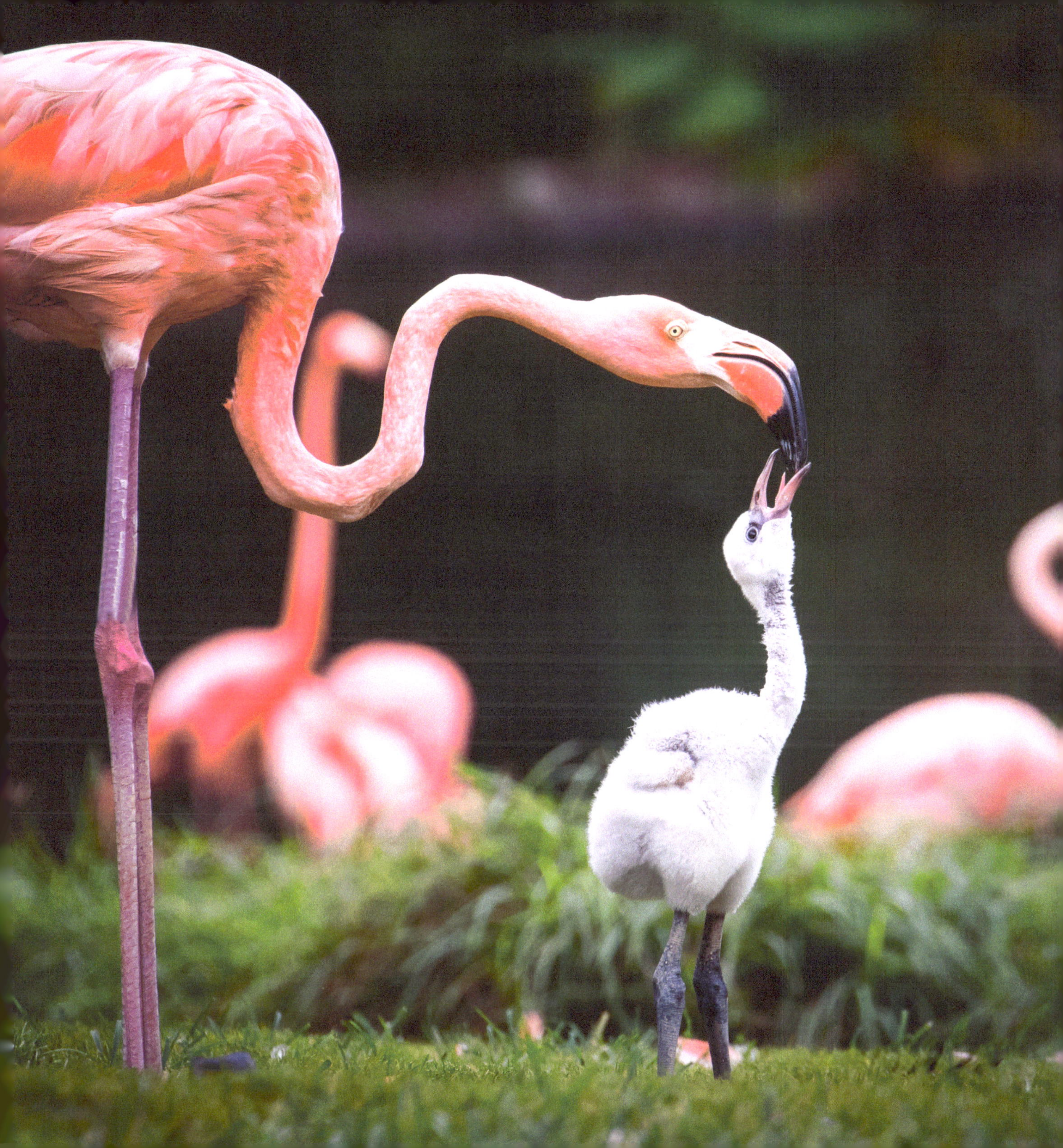

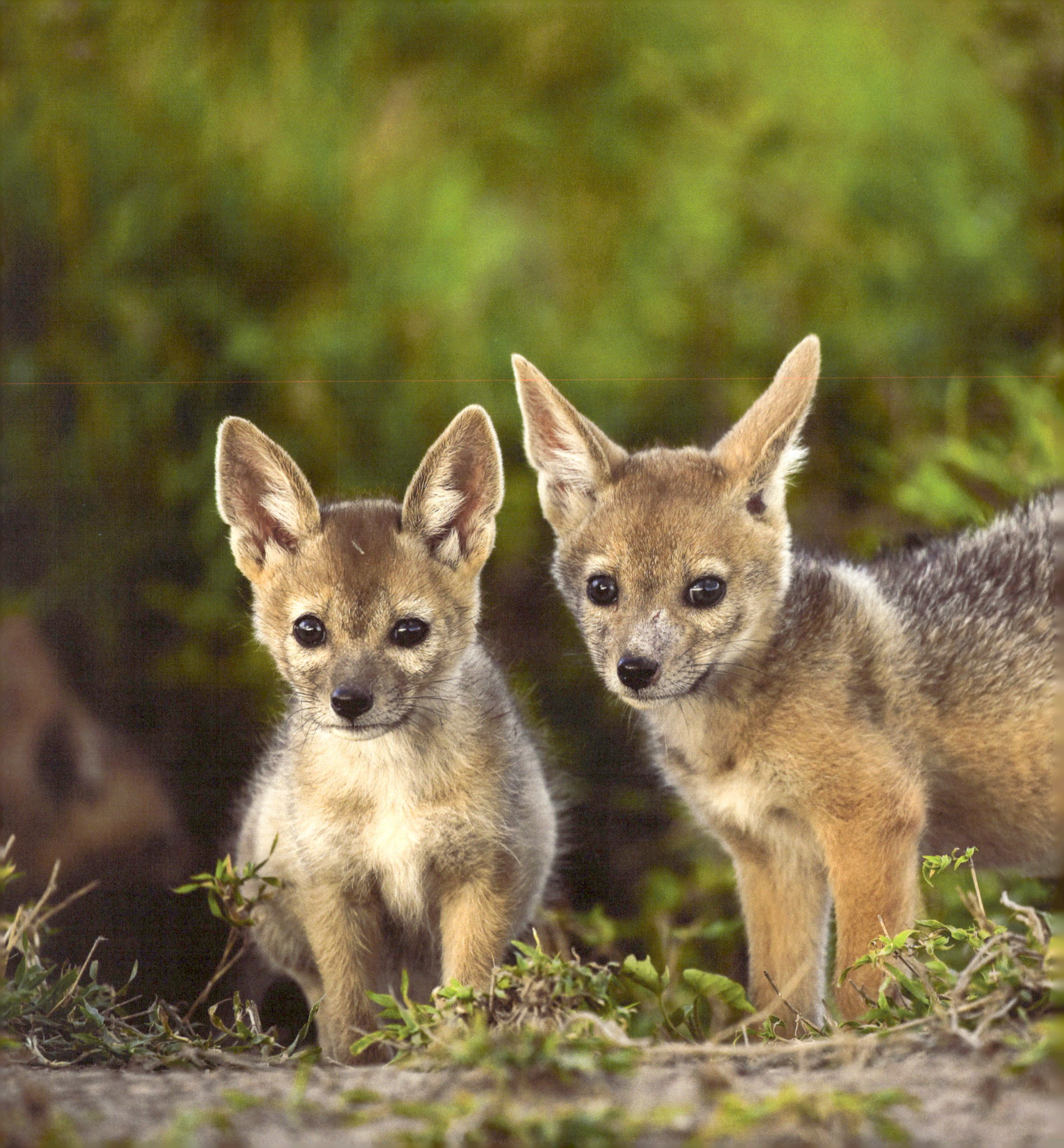

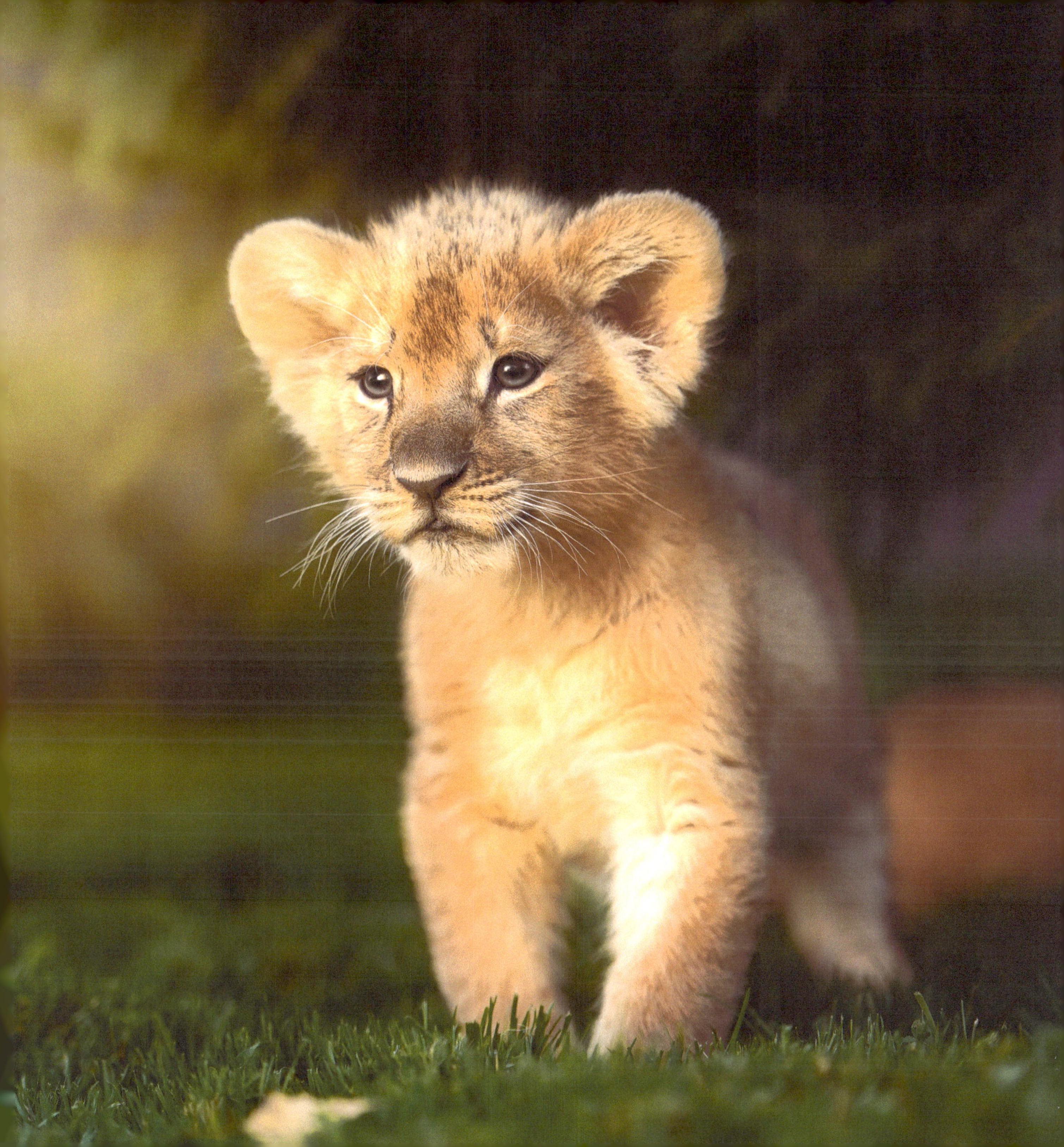

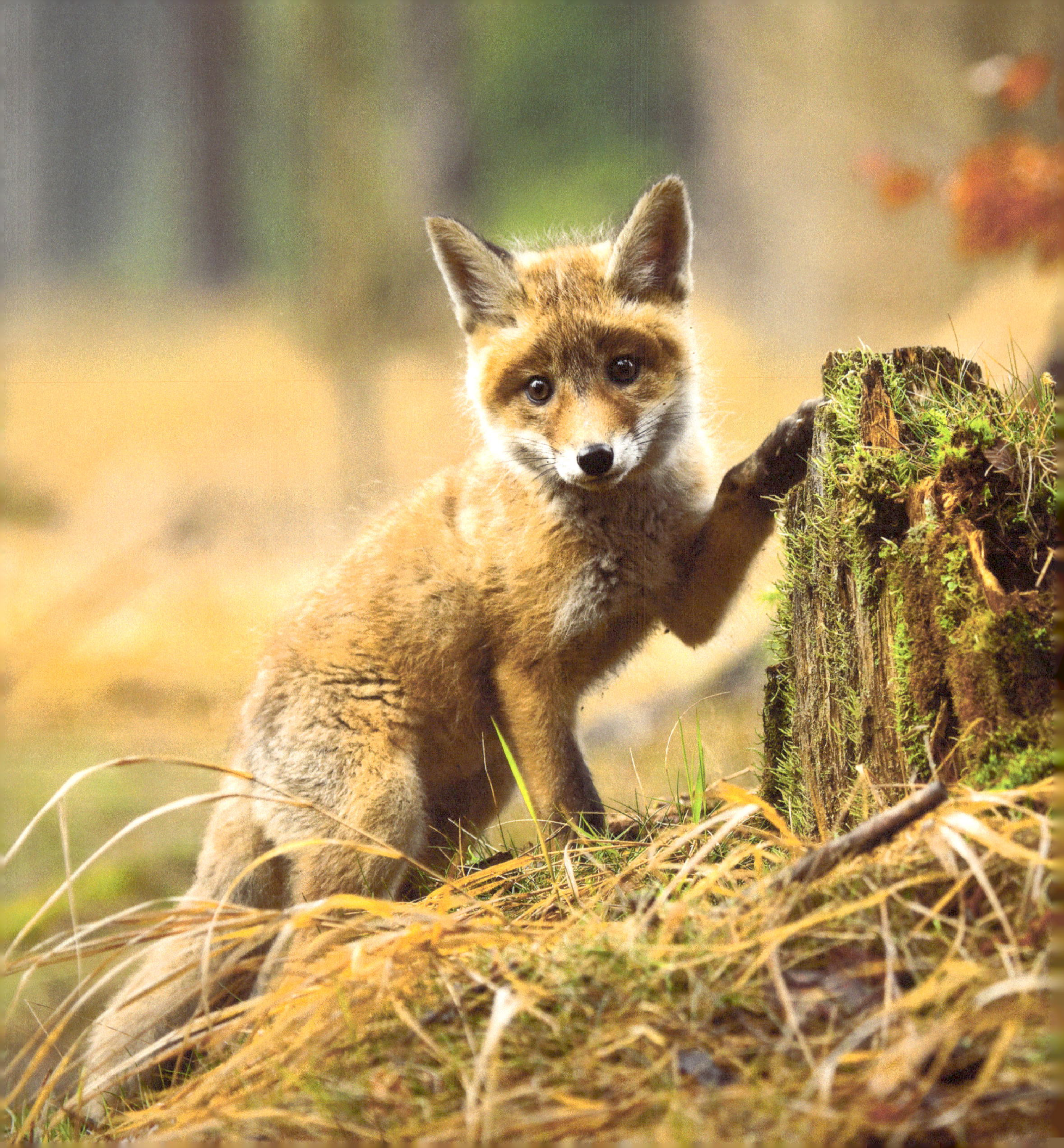

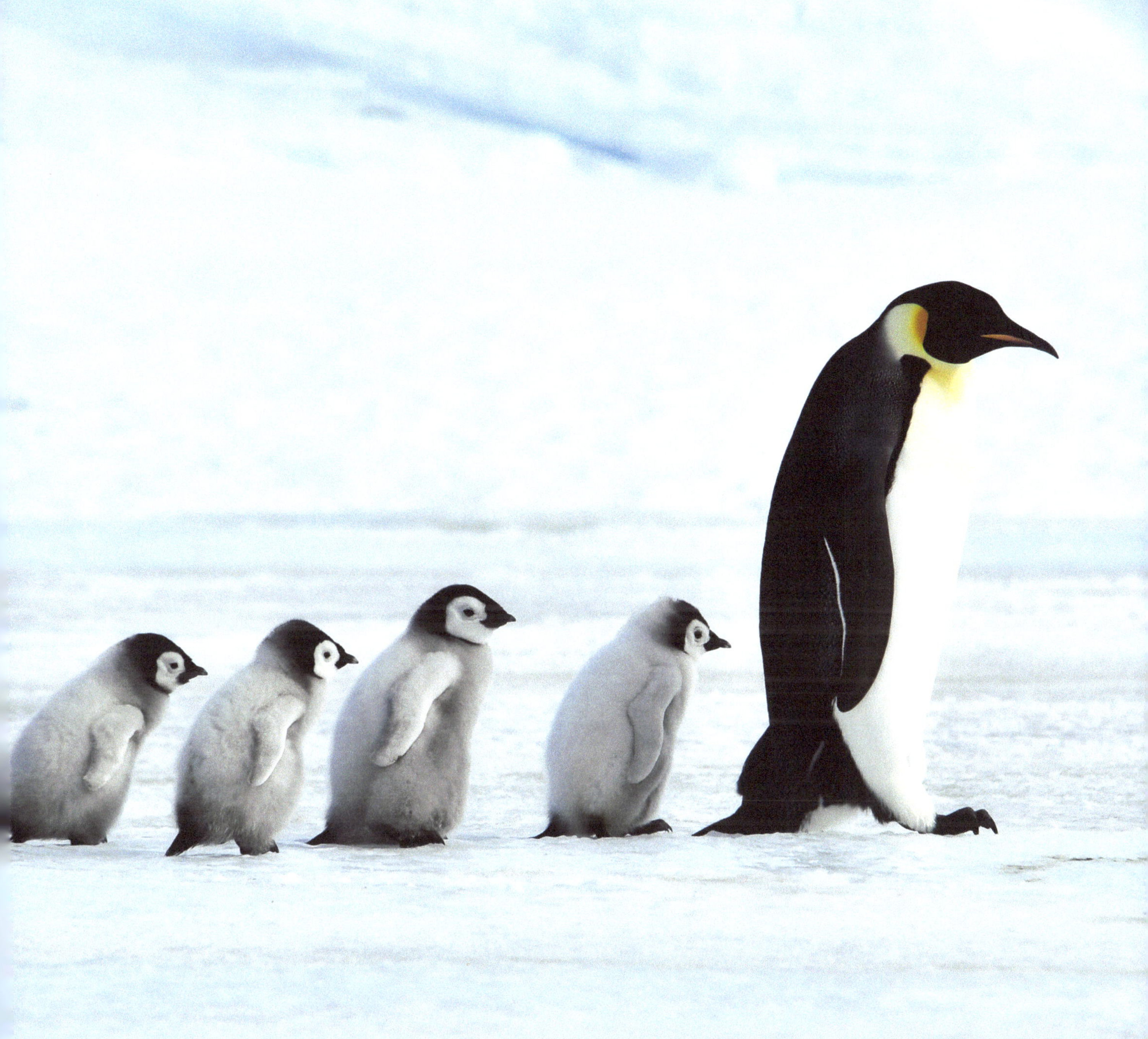

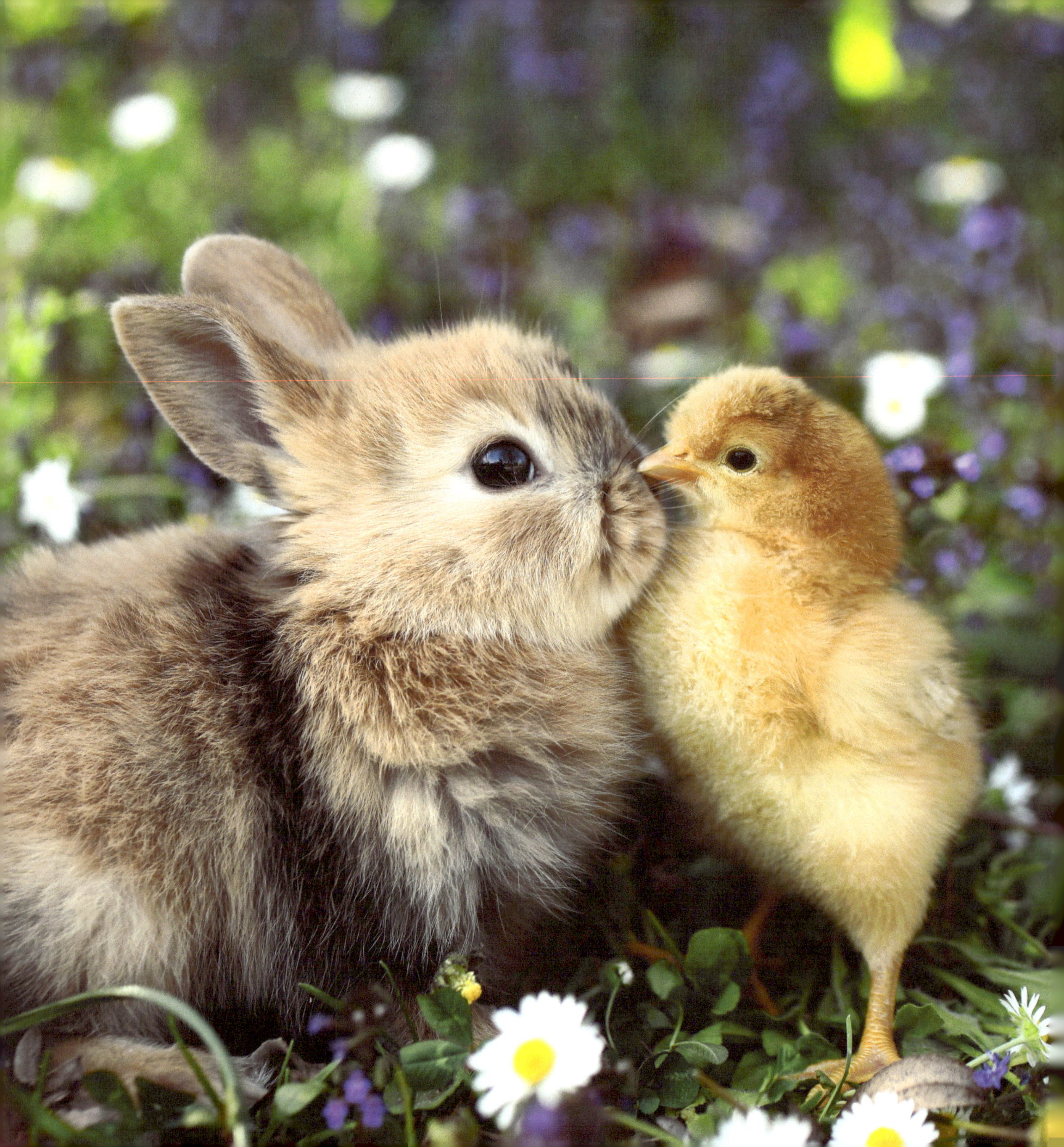

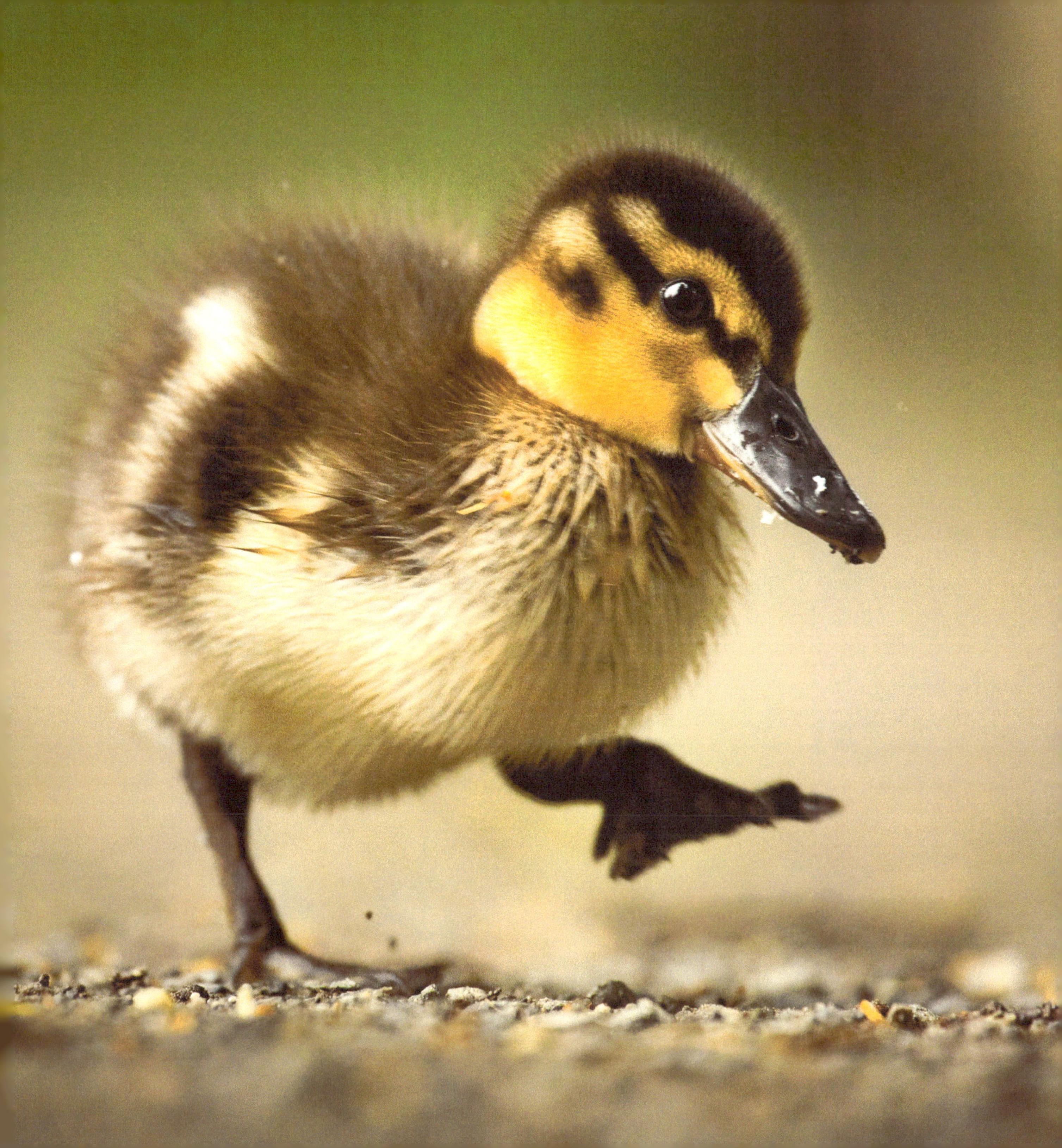

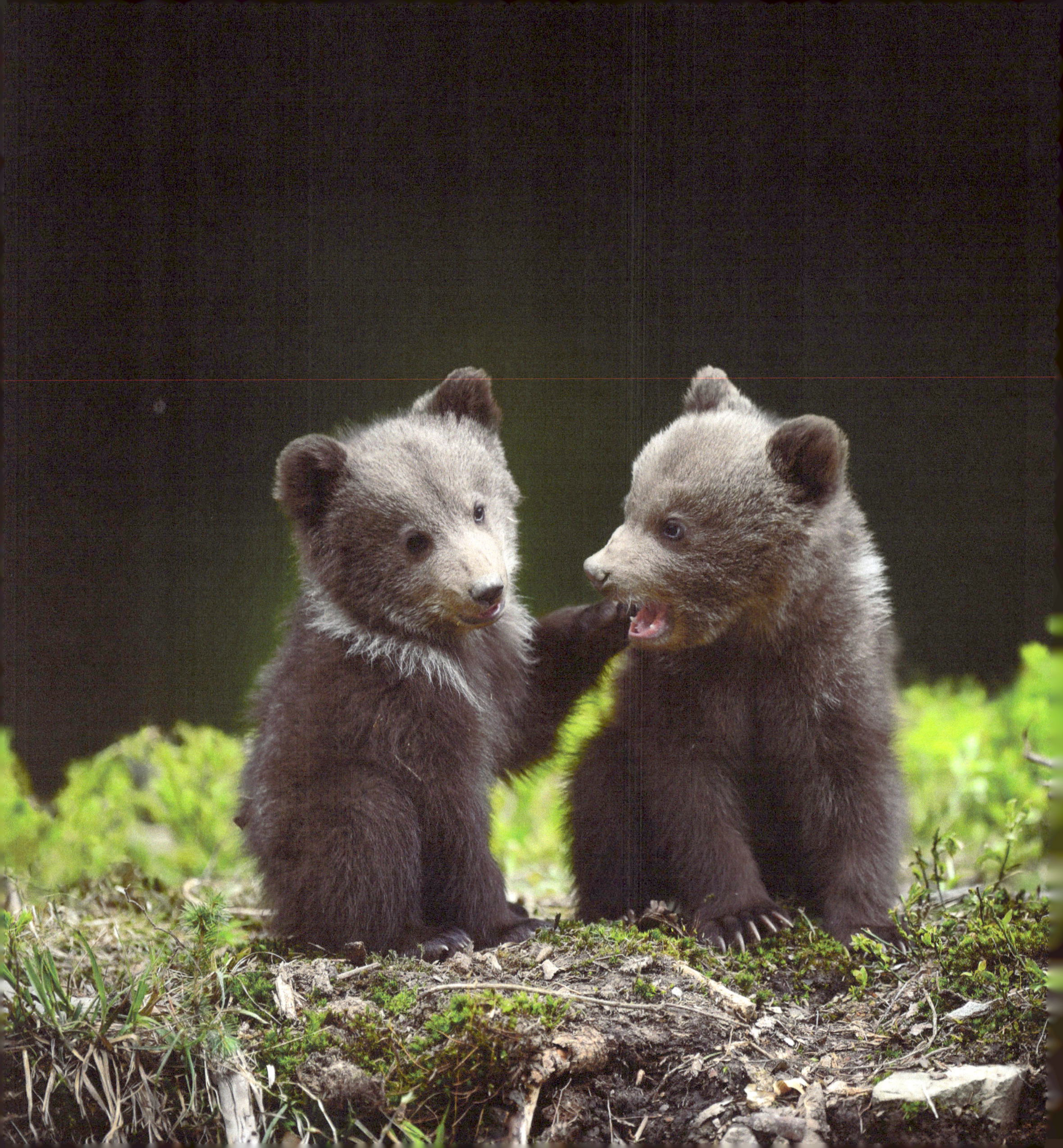

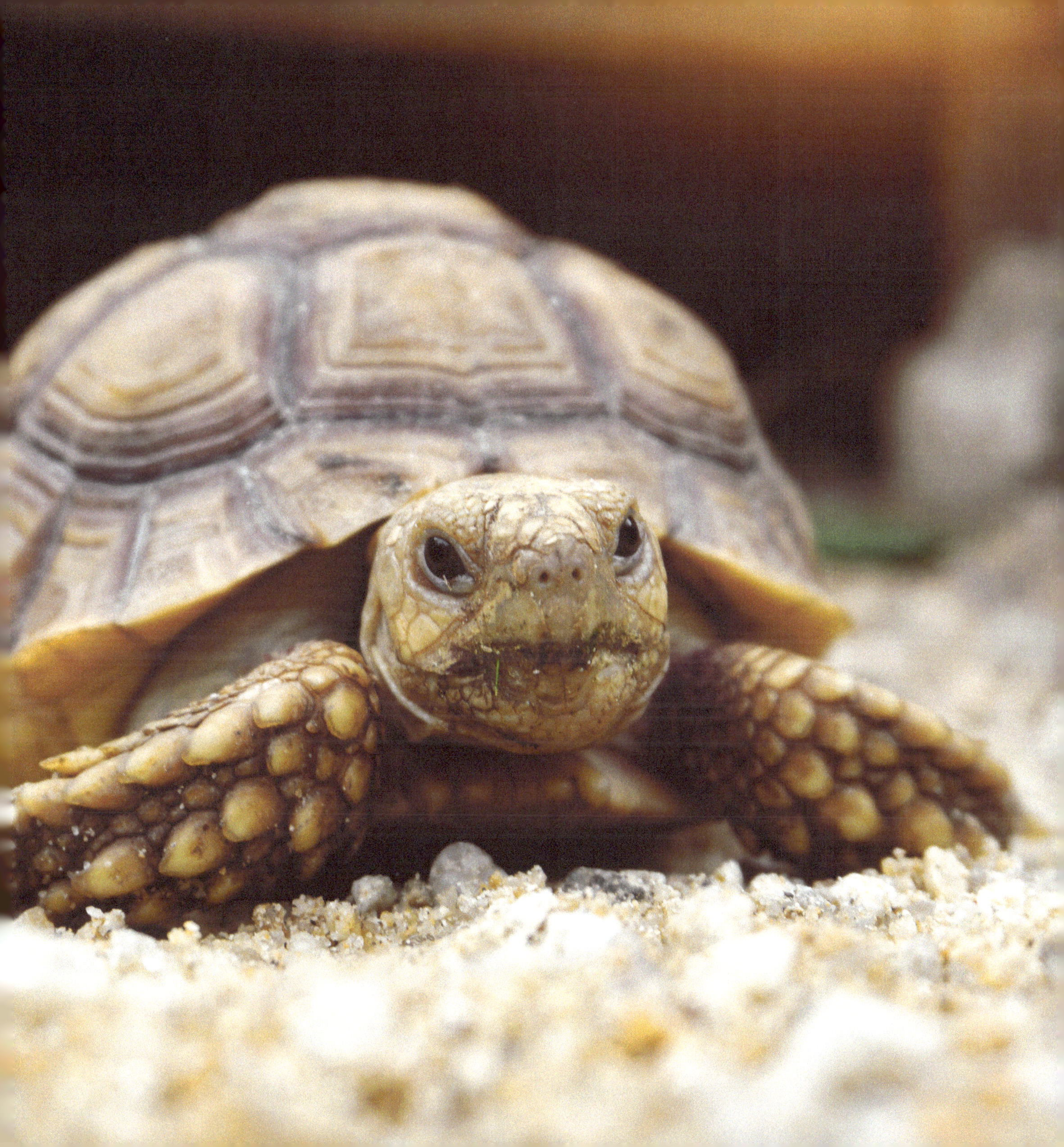

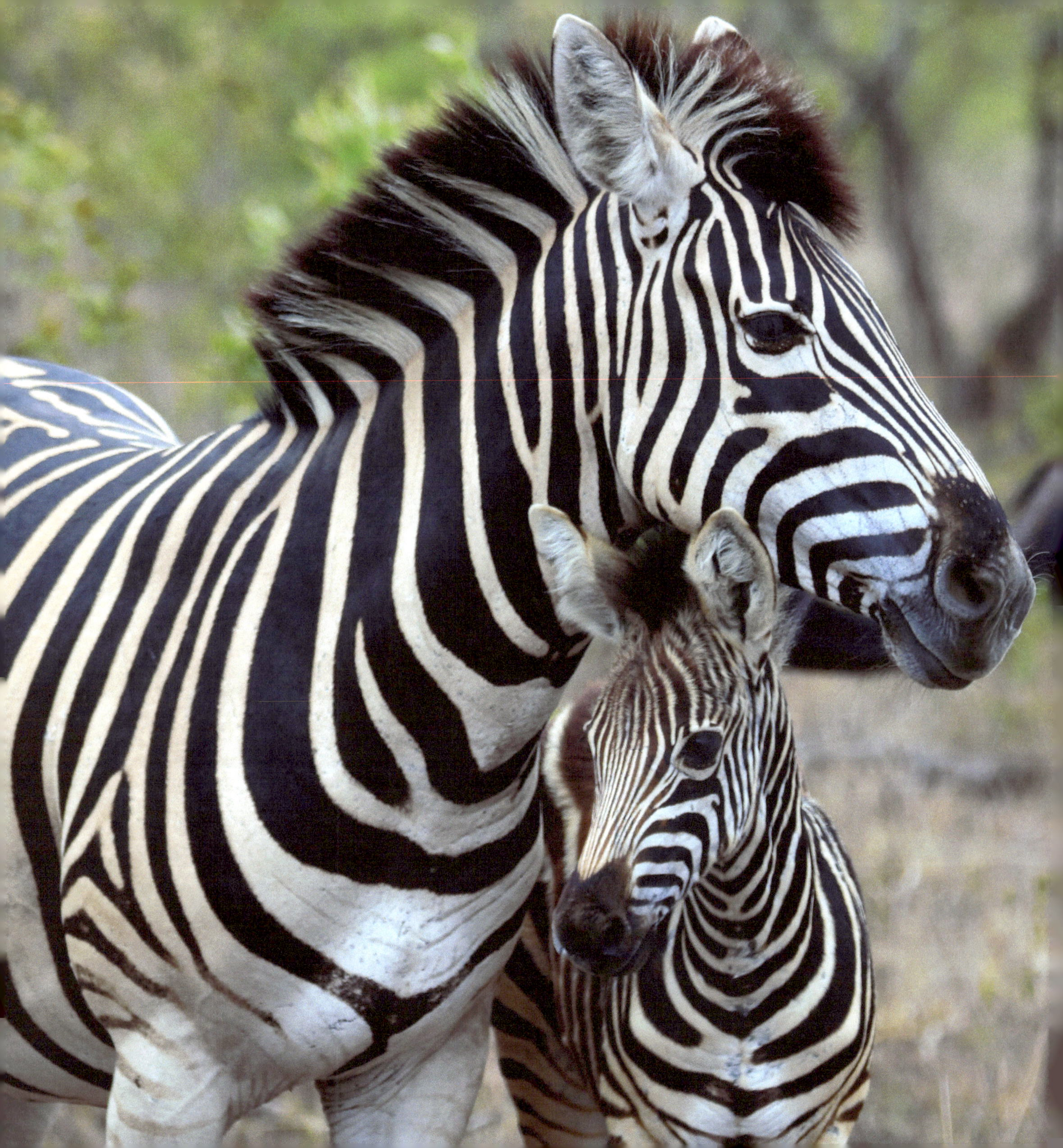

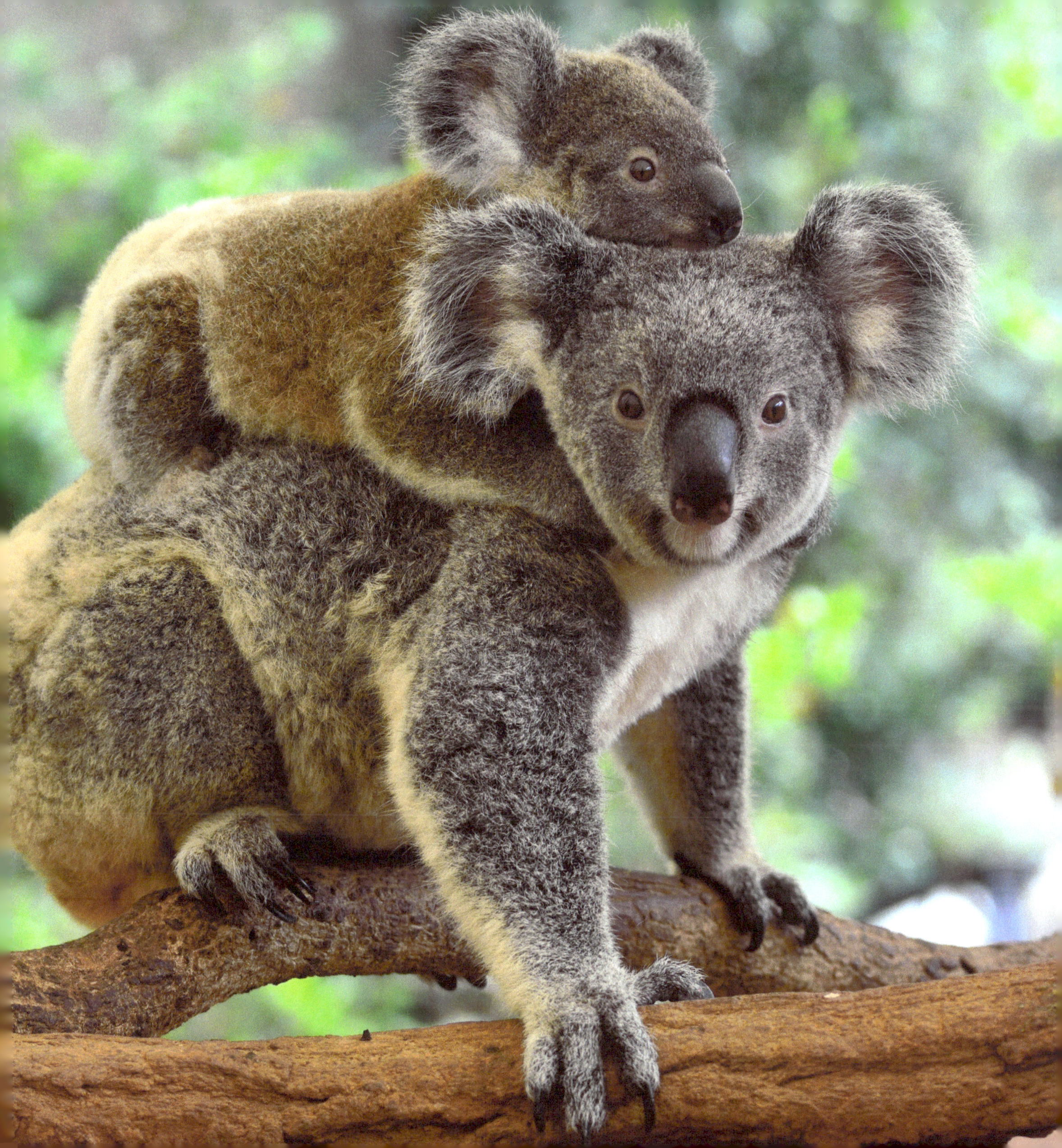

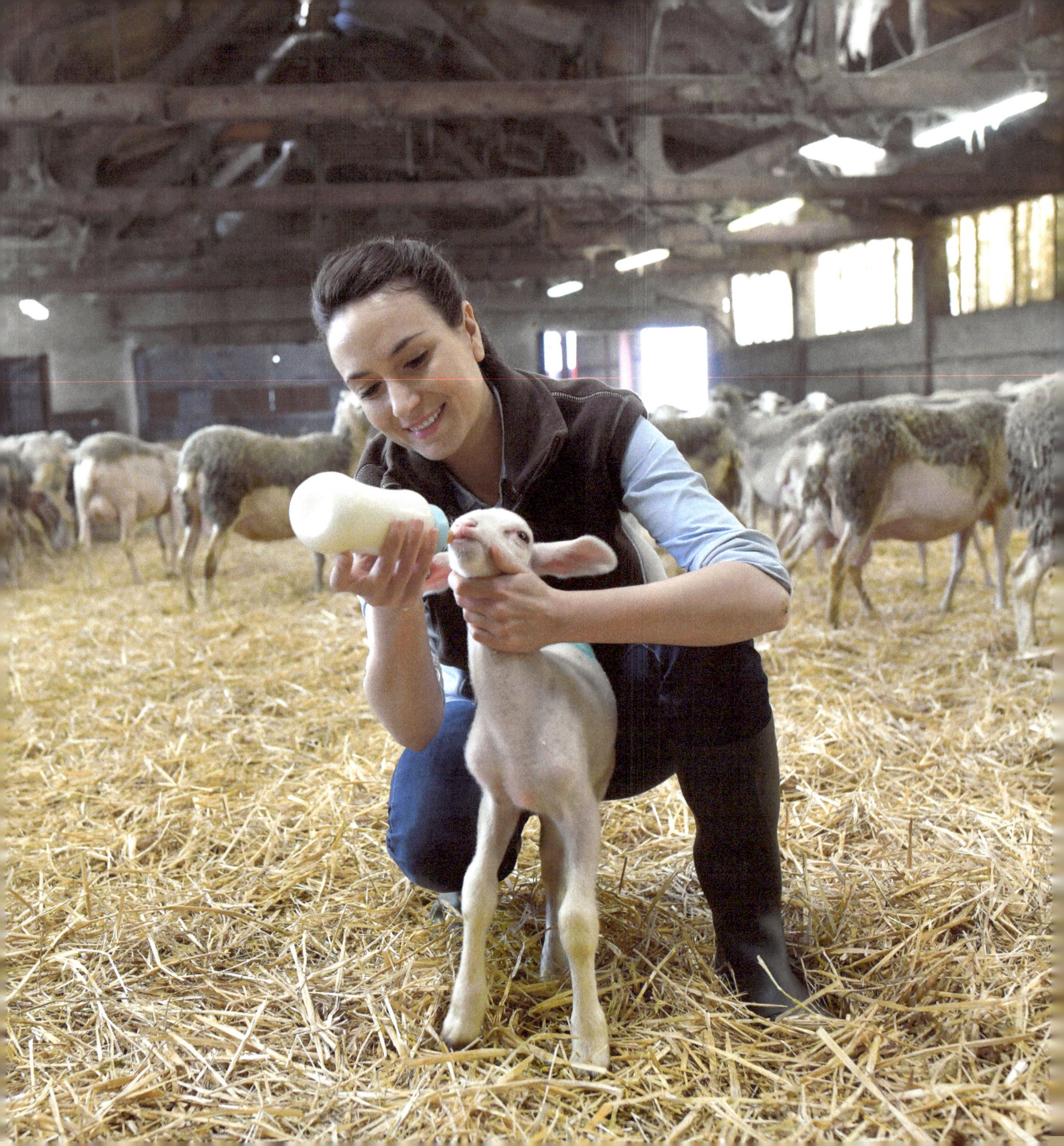

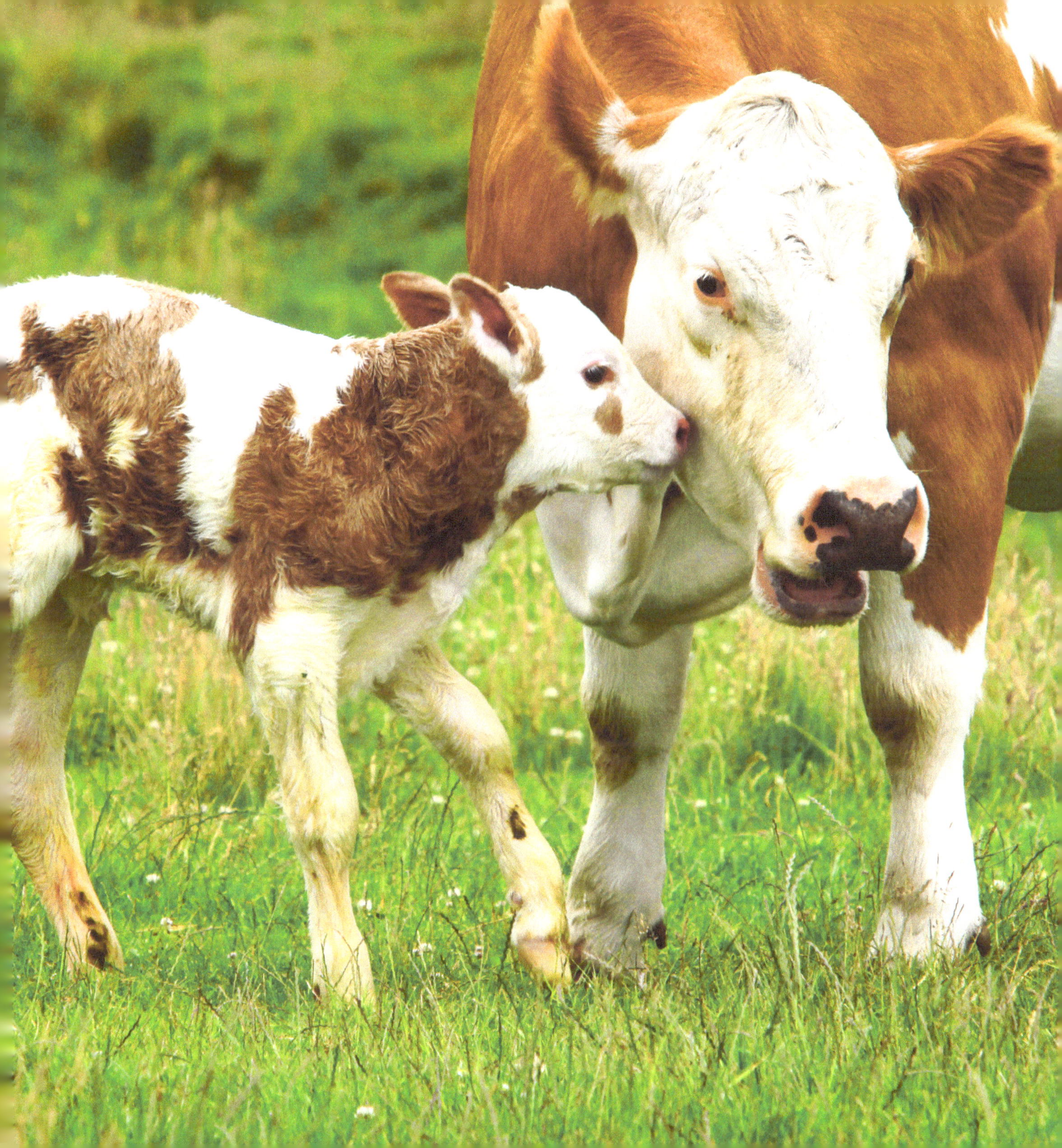

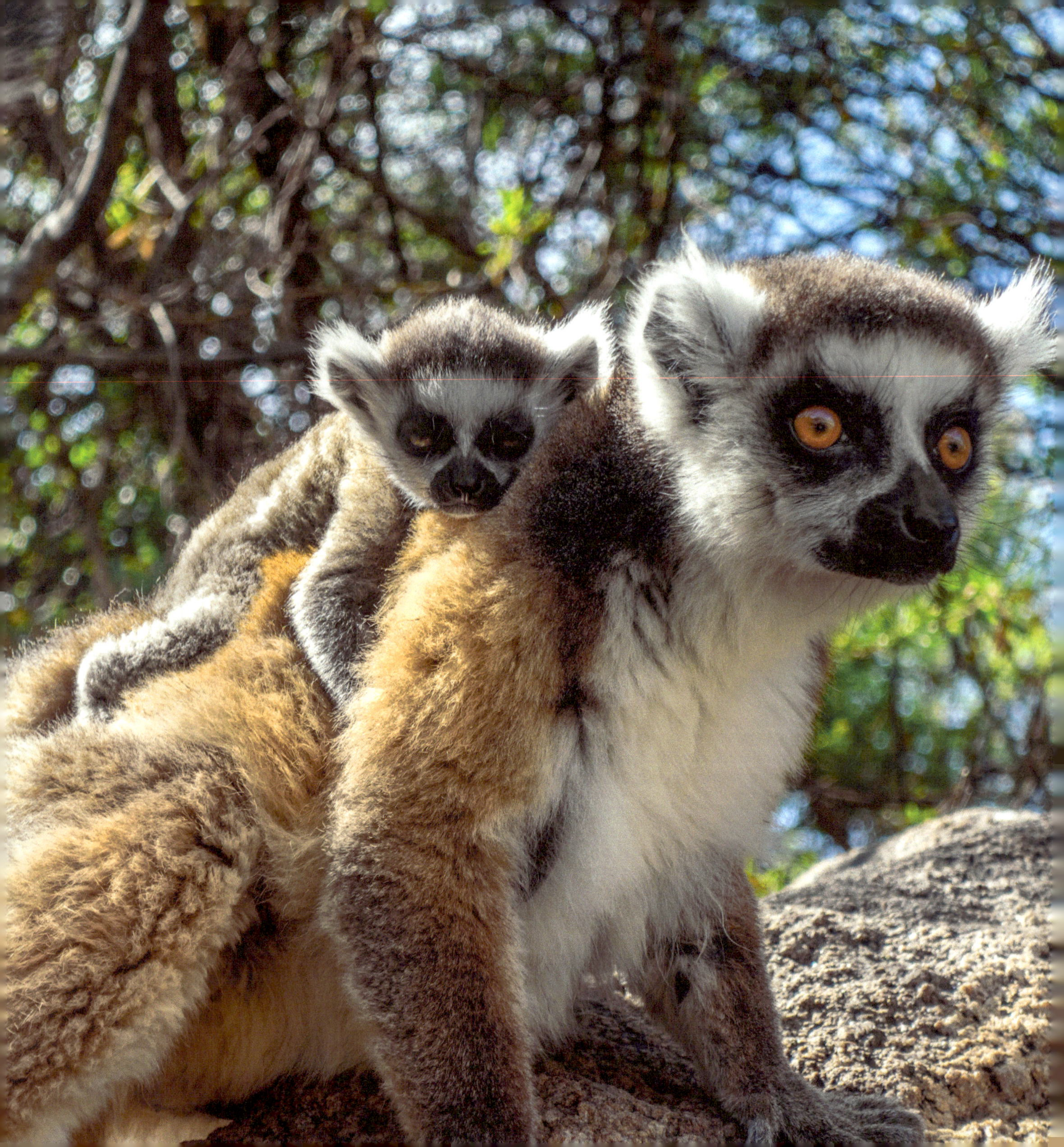

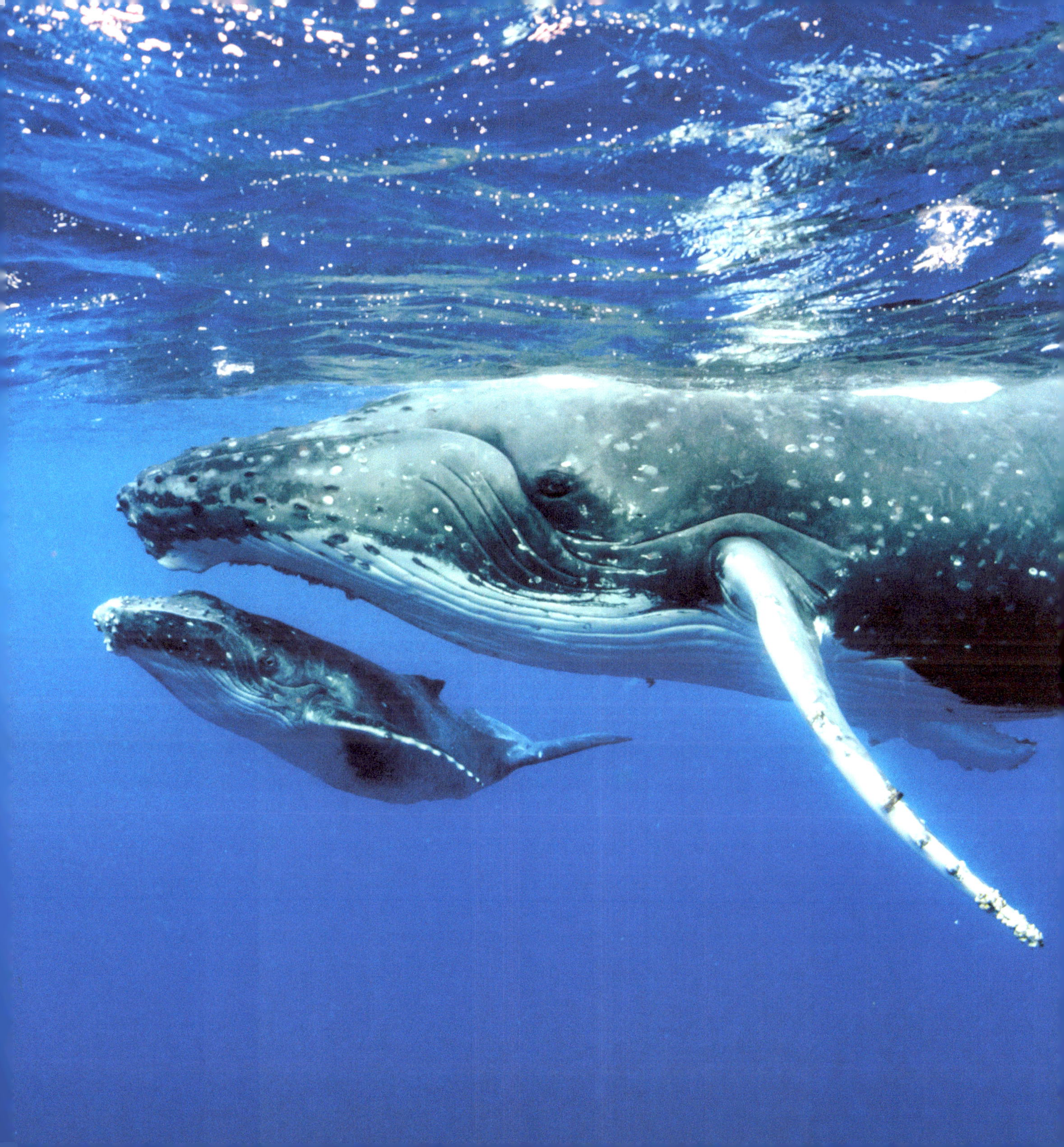

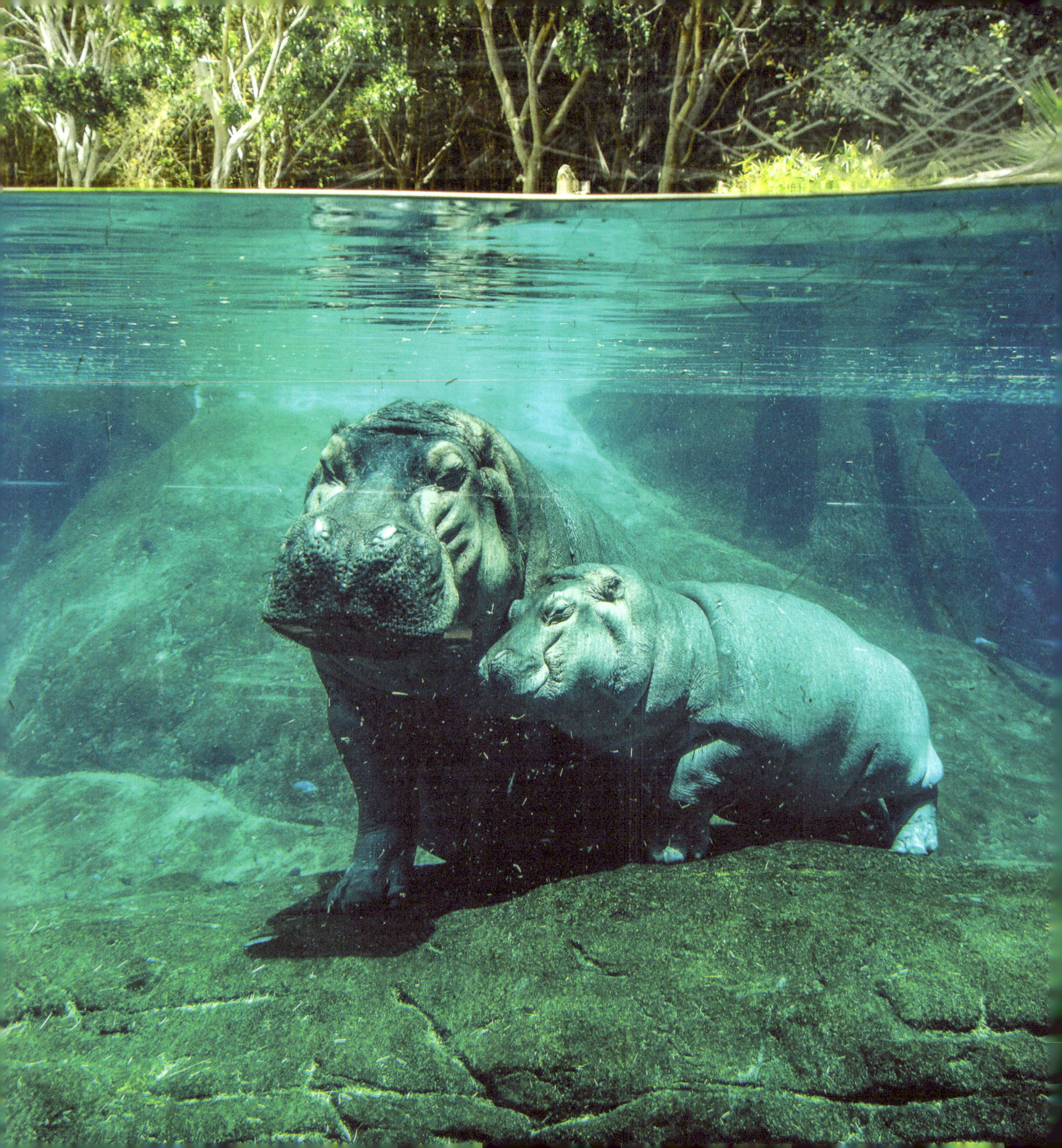

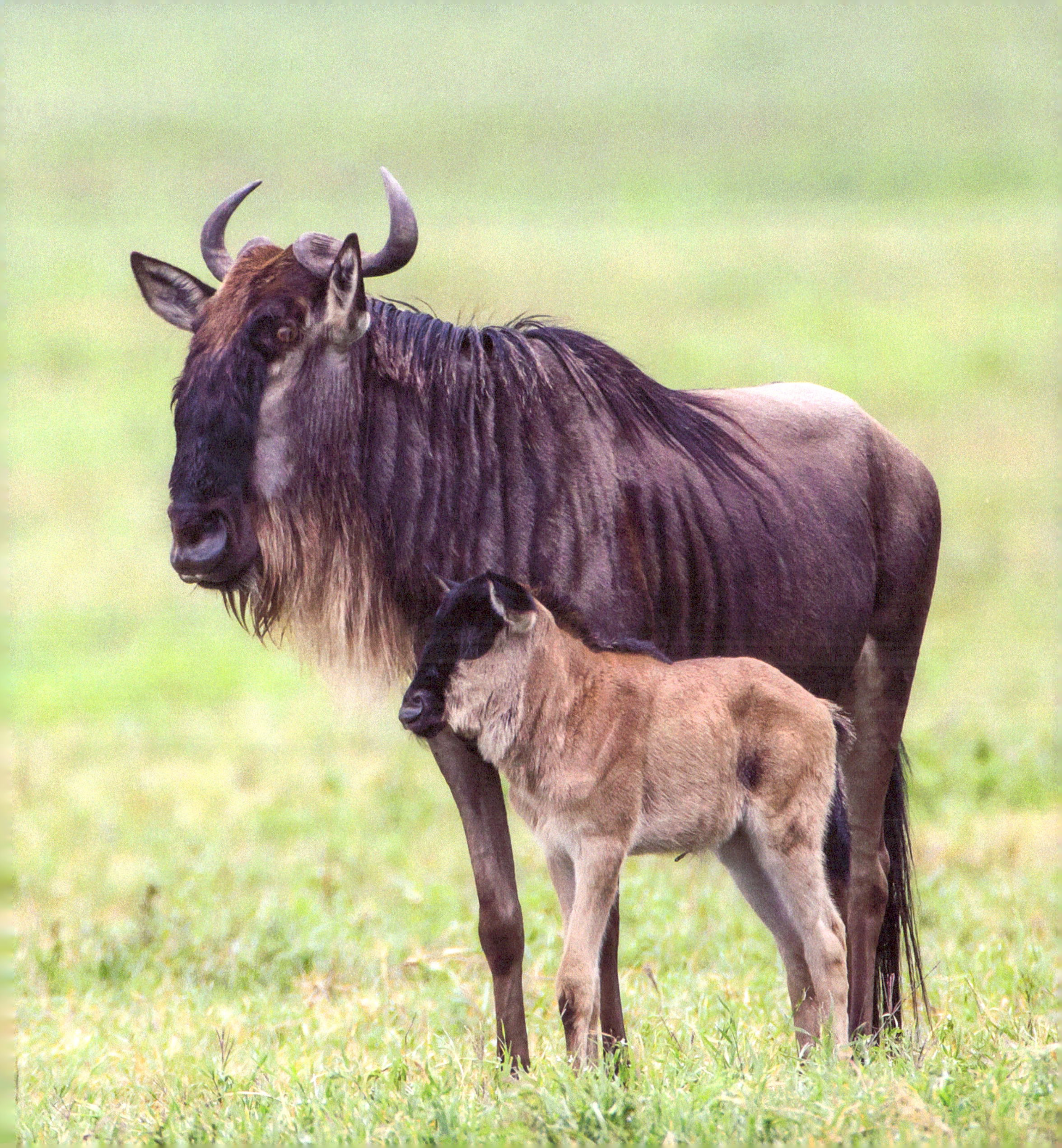

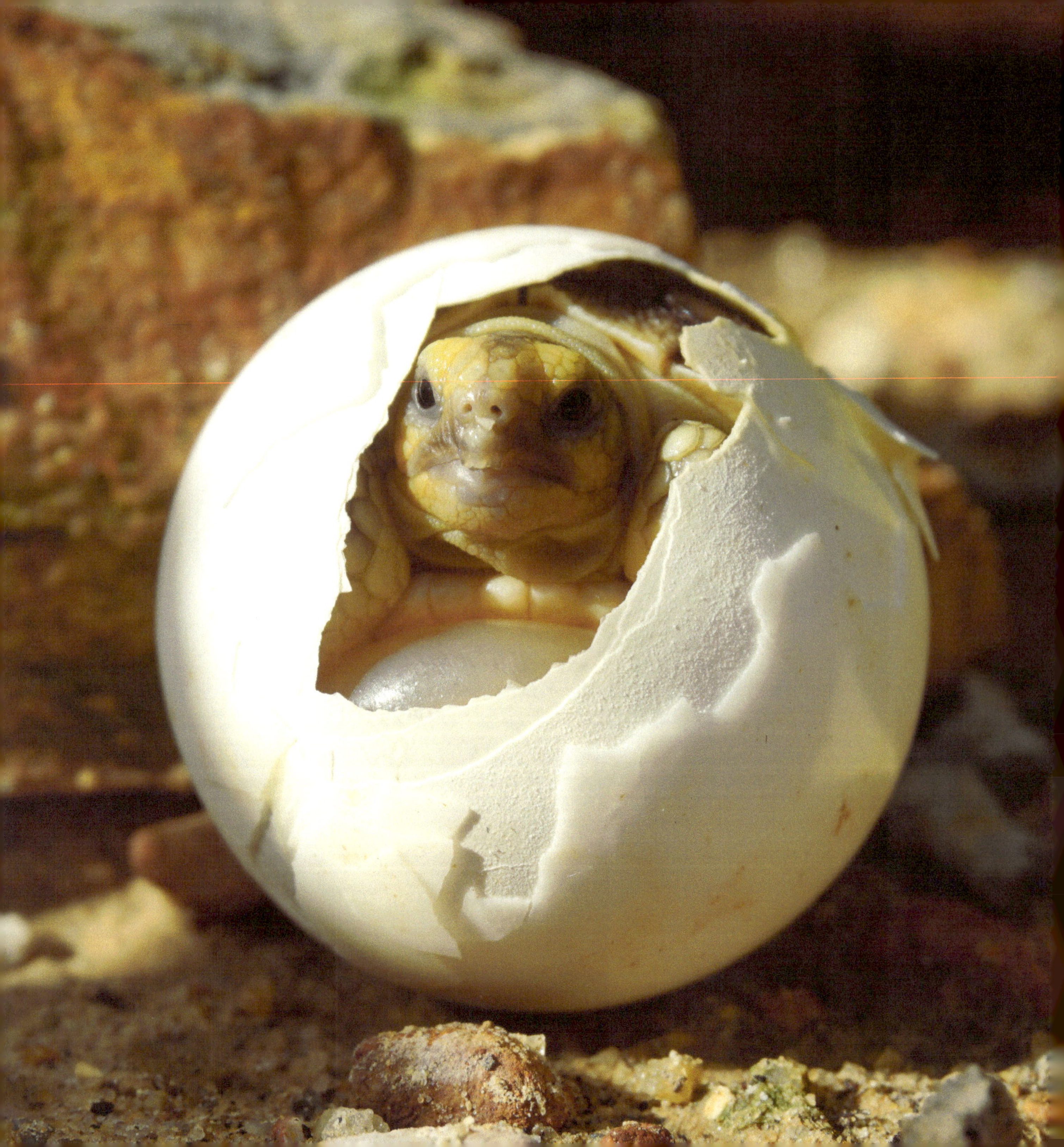

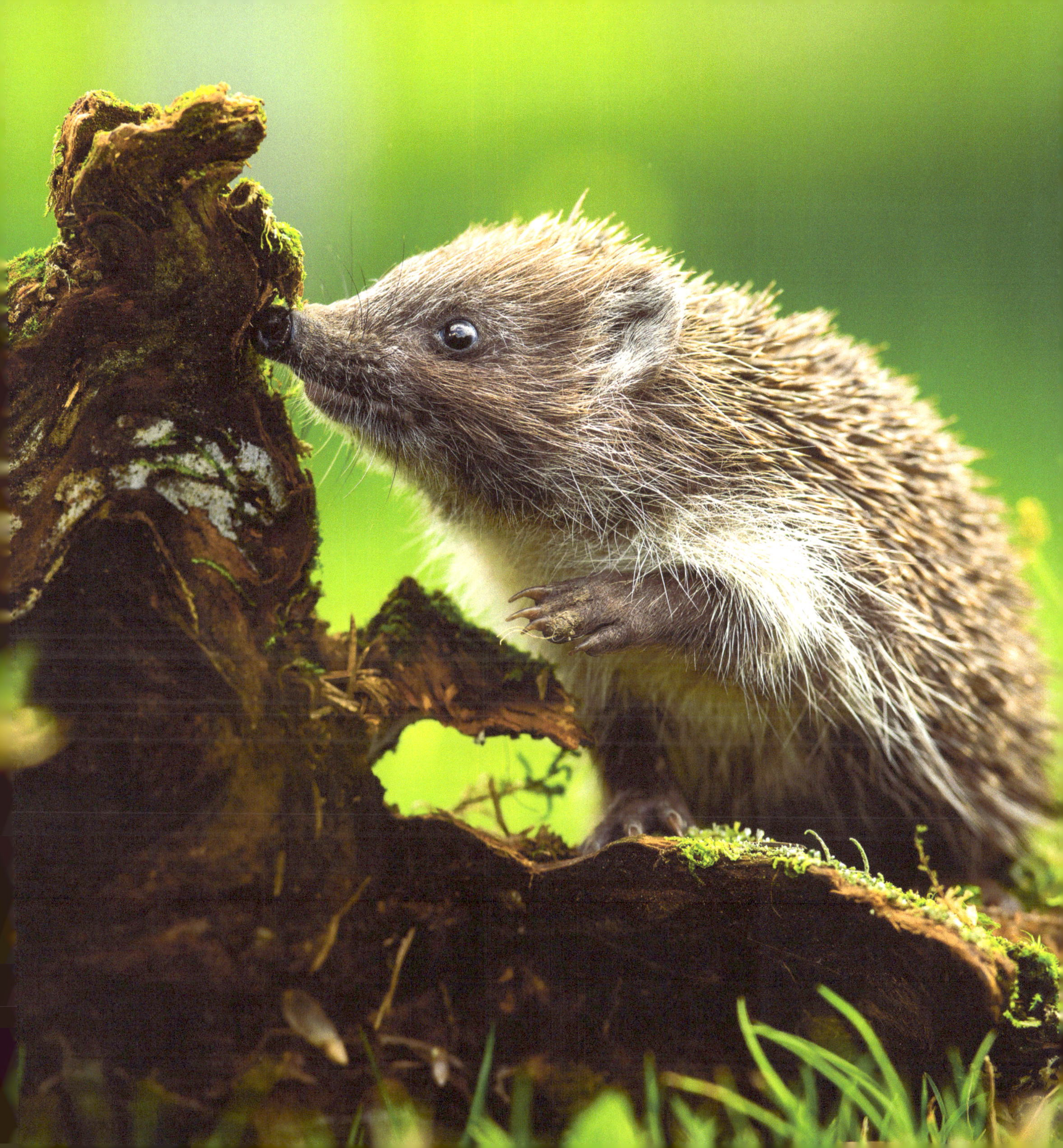

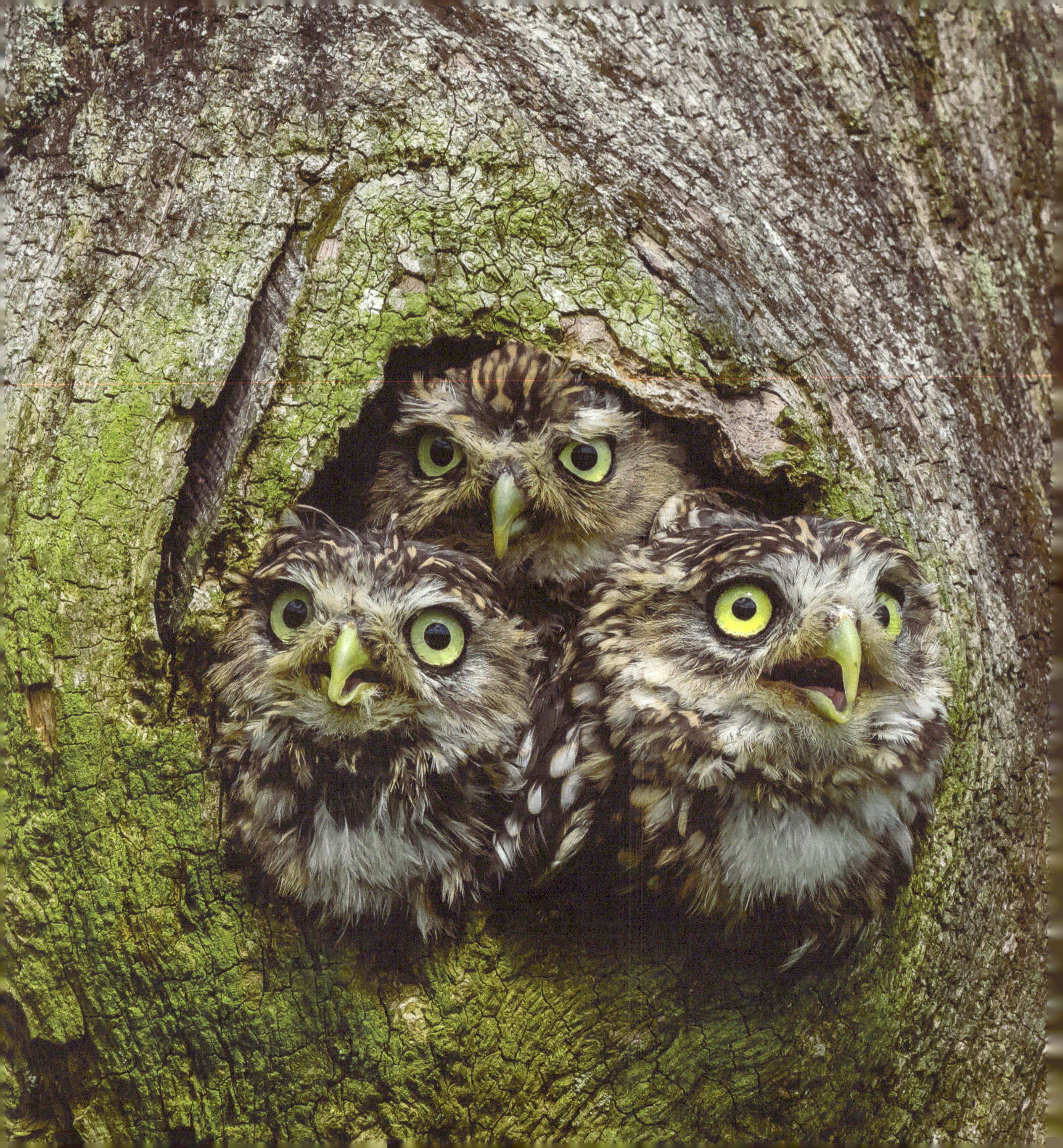

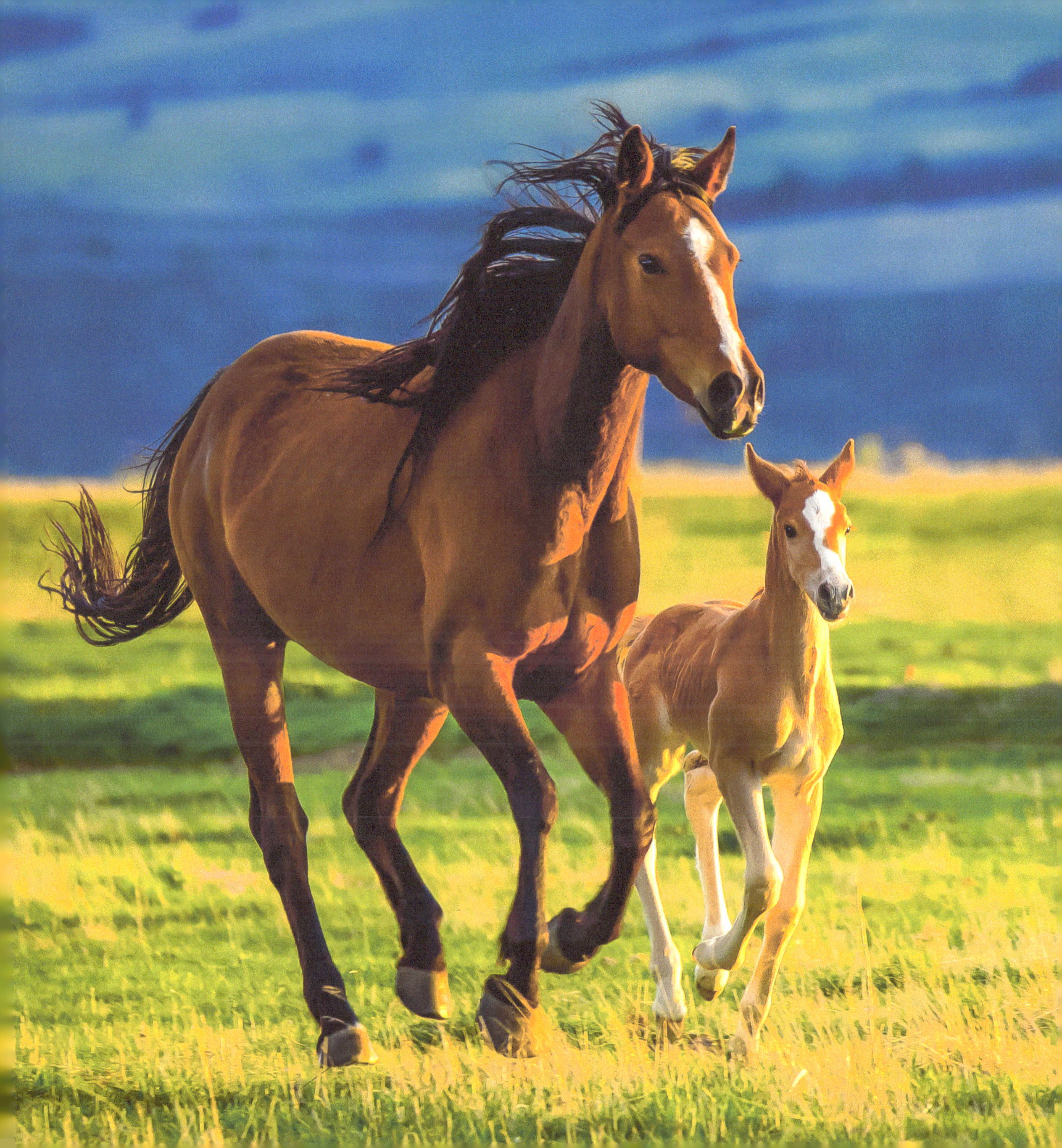

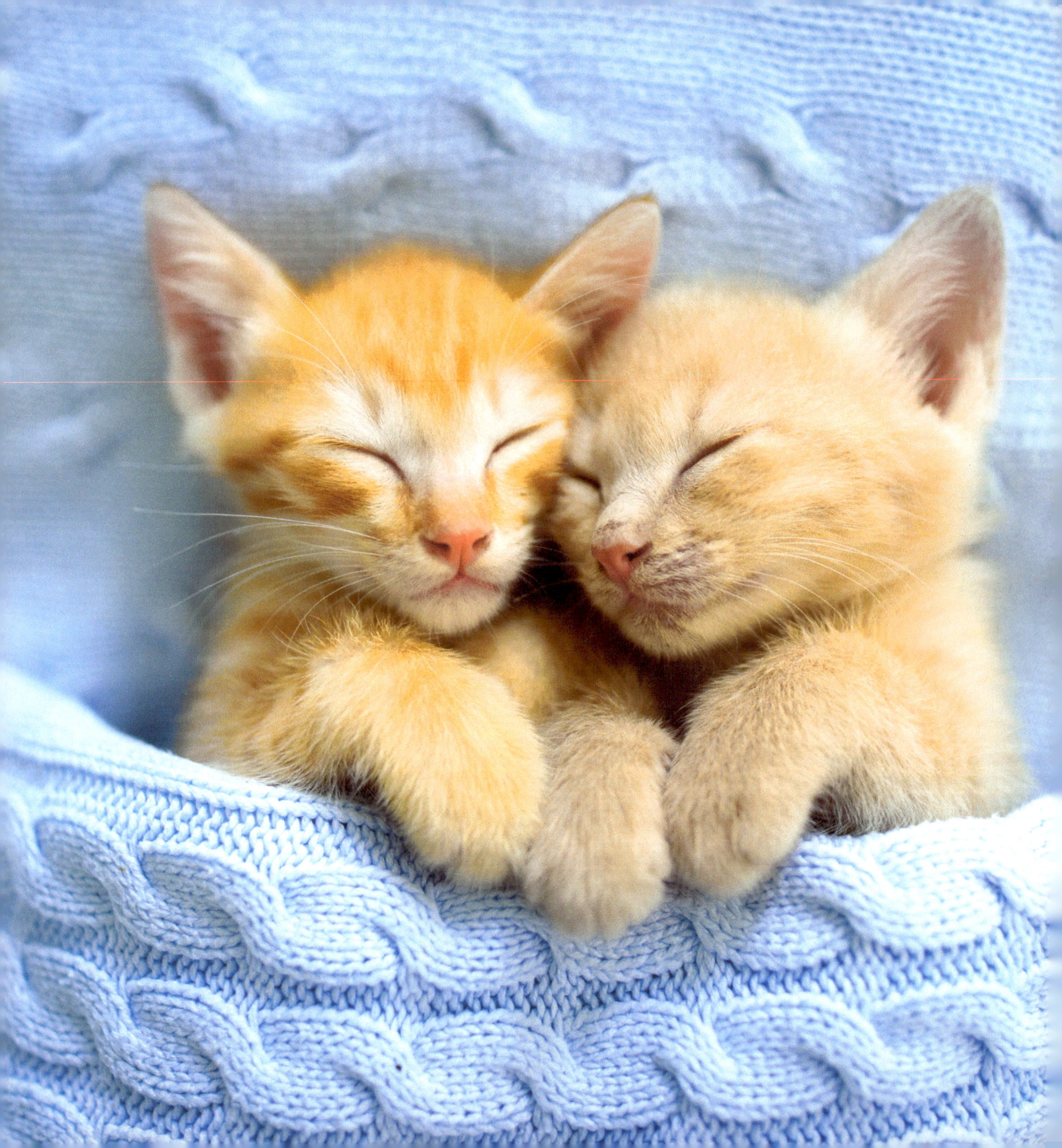

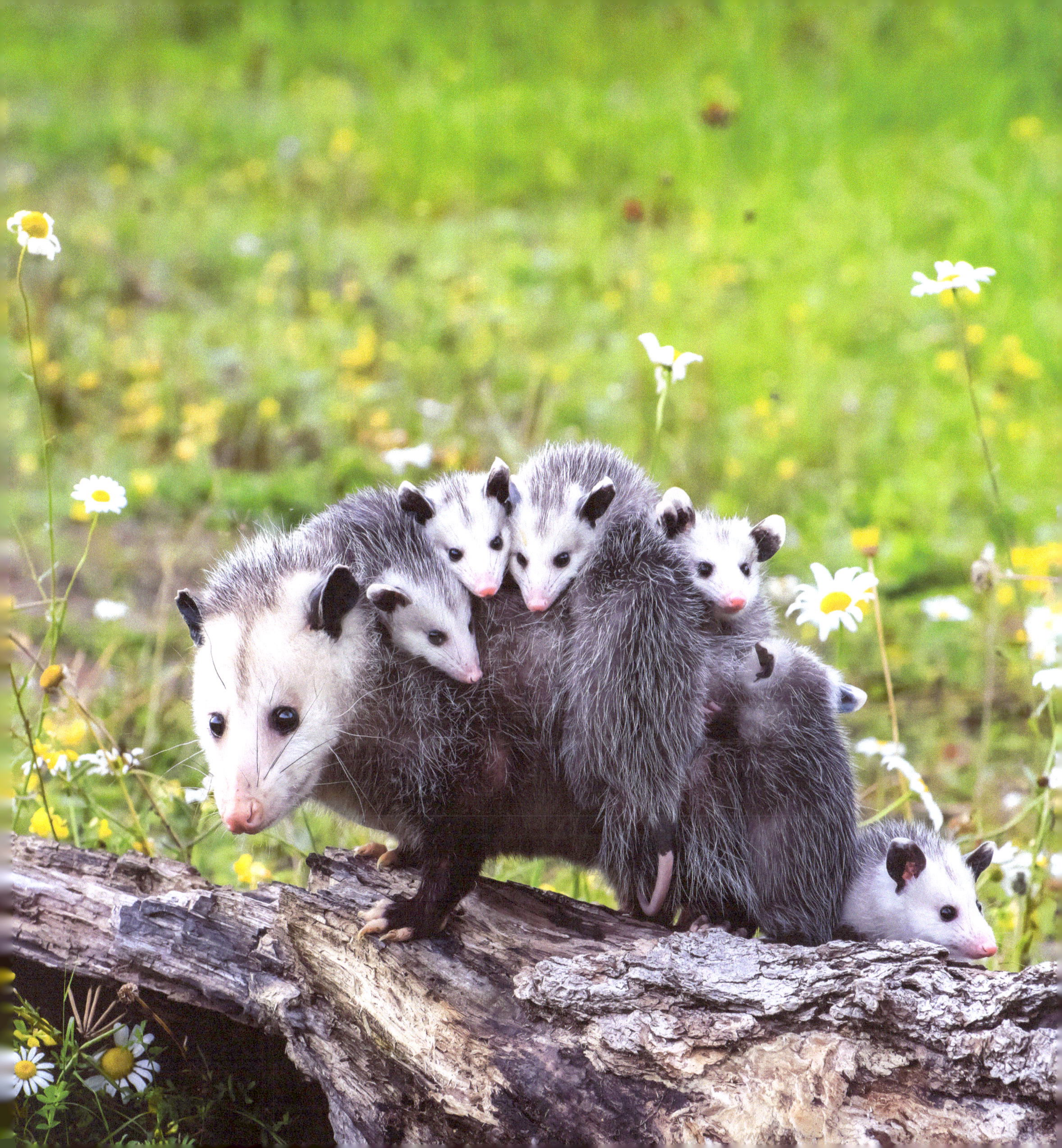

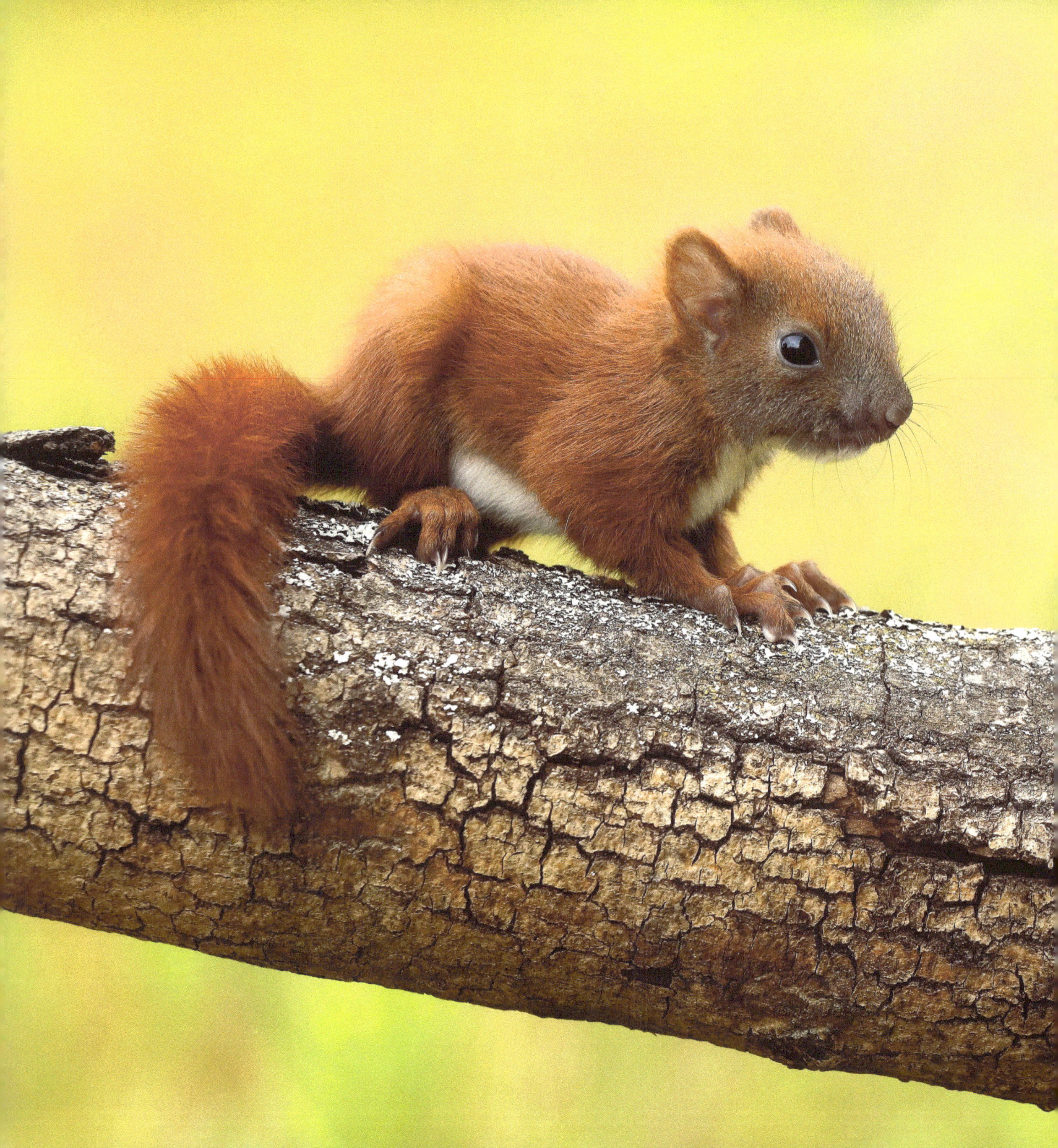

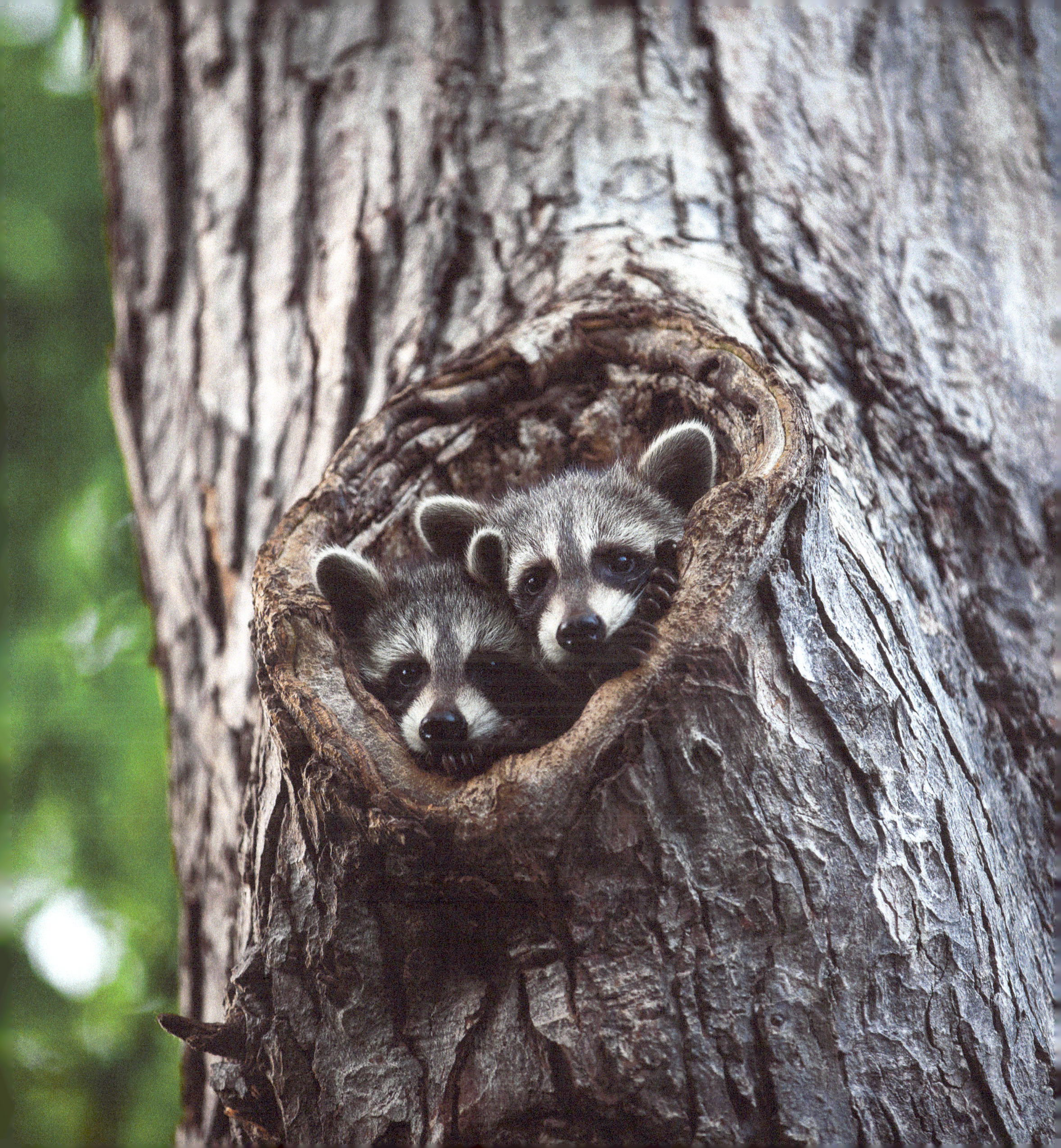

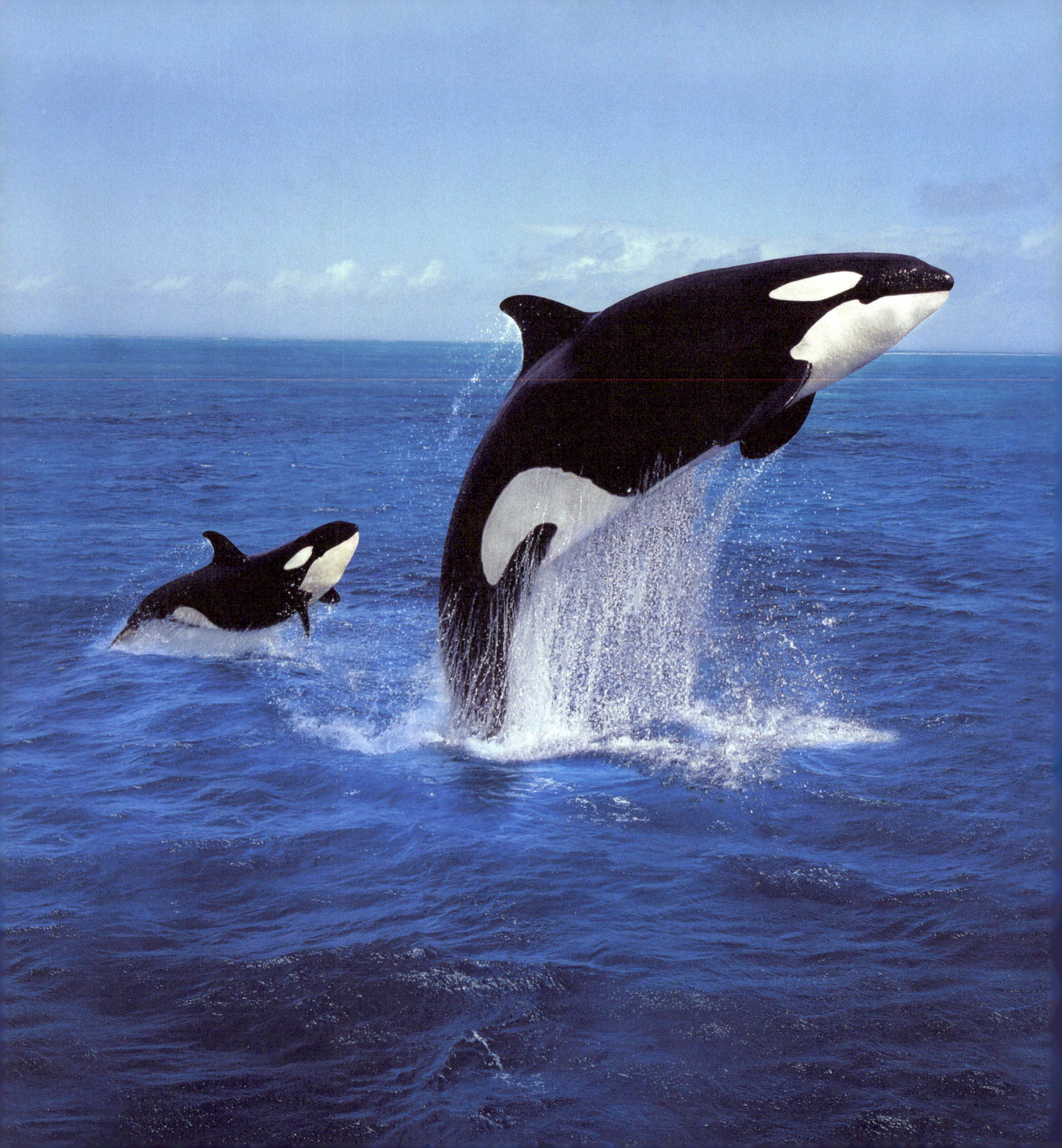

www.ingramcontent.com/pod-product-compliance
Lightning Source LLC
Chambersburg PA
CBHW042203030726
47602CB00007B/101